Novel Approaches to the Management of Sleep-Disordered Breathing

Editor

NEIL FREEDMAN

SLEEP MEDICINE CLINICS

www.sleep.theclinics.com

Consulting Editor
TEOFILO LEE-CHIONG Jr

June 2016 • Volume 11 • Number 2

ELSEVIER

1600 John F. Kennedy Boulevard • Suite 1800 • Philadelphia, Pennsylvania, 19103-2899

http://www.theclinics.com

SLEEP MEDICINE CLINICS Volume 11, Number 2
June 2016, ISSN 1556-407X, ISBN-13: 978-0-323-44634-1

Editor: Patrick Manley
Developmental Editor: Donald Mumford

Sleep Medicine Clinics (ISSN 1556-407X) is published quarterly by Elsevier Inc., 360 Park Avenue South, New York, NY 10010-1710. Months of issue are March, June, September and December. Business and Editorial Offices: 1600 John F. Kennedy Blvd., Ste. 1800, Philadelphia, PA 19103-2899. Customer Service Office: 3251 Riverport Lane, Maryland Heights, MO 63043. Periodicals postage paid at New York, NY and additional mailing offices. Subscription prices are $195.00 per year (US individuals), $100.00 (US students), $458.00 (US institutions), $235.00 (Canadian and international individuals), $135.00 (Canadian and international students), $519.00 (Canadian institutions) and $509.00 (International institutions). Foreign air speed delivery is included in all *Clinics* subscription prices. All prices are subject to change without notice. **POSTMASTER:** Send change of address to *Sleep Medicine Clinics*, Elsevier Health Sciences Division, Subscription Customer Service, 3251 Riverport Lane, Maryland Heights, MO 63043. Customer Service: **Tel: 1-800-654-2452 (U.S. and Canada); 314-447-8871 (outside U.S. and Canada). Fax: 314-447-8029. E-mail: journalscustomerservice-usa@elsevier.com (for print support); journalsonline support-usa@elsevier.com (for online support)**.

Reprints. For copies of 100 or more of articles in this publication, please contact the Commercial Reprints Department, Elsevier Inc., 360 Park Avenue South, New York, NY 10010-1710. Tel.: 212-633-3874; Fax: 212-633-3820; E-mail: reprints@elsevier.com.

Sleep Medicine Clinics is covered in *MEDLINE/PubMed (Index Medicus)*.

PROGRAM OBJECTIVE

The goal of *Sleep Clinics of North America* is to keep practicing physicians up to date with current clinical practice by providing timely articles reviewing the state of the art in patient care.

TARGET AUDIENCE

All practicing physicians and other healthcare professionals.

LEARNING OBJECTIVES

Upon completion of this activity, participants will be able to:

1. Review the challenges associated with treating sleep disordered breathing.
2. Discuss the efficacy of novel surgical and pharmacologic therapies for obstructive sleep apnea.
3. Recognize new approaches to the treatment of central sleep apnea.

ACCREDITATION

The Elsevier Office of Continuing Medical Education (EOCME) is accredited by the Accreditation Council for Continuing Medical Education (ACCME) to provide continuing medical education for physicians.

The EOCME designates this enduring material for a maximum of 15 *AMA PRA Category 1 Credit*(s)™. Physicians should claim only the credit commensurate with the extent of their participation in the activity.

All other health care professionals requesting continuing education credit for this enduring material will be issued a certificate of participation.

DISCLOSURE OF CONFLICTS OF INTEREST

The EOCME assesses conflict of interest with its instructors, faculty, planners, and other individuals who are in a position to control the content of CME activities. All relevant conflicts of interest that are identified are thoroughly vetted by EOCME for fair balance, scientific objectivity, and patient care recommendations. EOCME is committed to providing its learners with CME activities that promote improvements or quality in healthcare and not a specific proprietary business or a commercial interest.

The planning committee, staff, authors and editors listed below have identified no financial relationships or relationships to products or devices they or their spouse/life partner have with commercial interest related to the content of this CME activity:

Rohit Budhiraja, MD; Anjali Fortna; Neil Freedman, MD; Alex Gileles-Hillel, MD; David Gozal, MD, MBA; Dennis Hwang, MD; Abdelnaby Khalyfa, PhD; Matthew Kim, MD; Tomasz J. Kuźniar, MD, PhD, FCCP, FAASM; Atul Malhotra, MD; Patrick Manley; Todd D. Morgan, DMD; Robert L. Owens, MD; Susan Redline, MD, MPH; Scott A. Sands, PhD; Erin Scheckenbach; Ronaldo A. Sevilla Berrios, MD; Rajakumar Venkatesan.

The planning committee, staff, authors and editors listed below have identified financial relationships or relationships to products or devices they or their spouse/life partner have with commercial interest related to the content of this CME activity:

Peter C. Gay, MD has research support from Fisher & Paykel Appliances Limited.

Robin Germany, MD has an employment affiliation with Respicardia, Inc.

John J. Greer, PhD is a consultant/advisor for, with stock ownership in, and receives royalties/patents from, RespireRx Pharmaceuticals Inc.

Shahrokh Javaheri, MD is on the speakers' bureau for Koninklijke Philips N.V. and ResMed, and is a consultant/advisor for Respicardia, Inc. and LivaNova PLC.

Teofilo Lee-Chiong Jr, MD has stock ownership in, research support from, and an employment affiliation with Koninklijke Philips N.V., is a consultant/advisor for CareCore National and Elsevier B.V.; and has royalties/patents with Elsevier B.V.; Lippincott; John Wiley & Sons, Inc.; Oxford University Press; and CreateSpace, a DBA of On-Demand Publishing, LLC.

Ryan J. Soose, MD is a consultant/advisor for, with research support from, Inspire Medical Systems, Inc.

Robert Thomas, MD, MMSc is a consultant/advisor for Garson Lehrman Group, Inc., has research support from Medical Depot, Inc. dba Drive DeVilbiss Healthcare, and receives royalties/patents from MyCardio, LLC; Medical Depot, Inc. dba Drive DeVilbiss Healthcare; and Beth Israel Deaconess Medical Center.

David P. White, MD is a consultant/advisor for Koninklijke Philips N.V. and NightBalance B.V., and has stock ownership in and an employment affiliation with ApniCure, Inc.

UNAPPROVED/OFF-LABEL USE DISCLOSURE

The EOCME requires CME faculty to disclose to the participants:

1. When products or procedures being discussed are off-label, unlabelled, experimental, and/or investigational (not US Food and Drug Administration [FDA] approved); and
2. Any limitations on the information presented, such as data that are preliminary or that represent ongoing research, interim analyses, and/or unsupported opinions. Faculty may discuss information about pharmaceutical agents that is outside of FDA-approved labelling. This information is intended solely for CME and is not intended to promote off-label use of these

medications. If you have any questions, contact the medical affairs department of the manufacturer for the most recent prescribing information.

TO ENROLL
To enroll in the Sleep Medicines Clinic Continuing Medical Education program, call customer service at 1-800-654-2452 or sign up online at http://www.theclinics.com/home/cme. The CME program is available to subscribers for an additional annual fee of USD $140.

METHOD OF PARTICIPATION
In order to claim credit, participants must complete the following:
1. Complete enrolment as indicated above.
2. Read the activity.
3. Complete the CME Test and Evaluation. Participants must achieve a score of 70% on the test. All CME Tests and Evaluations must be completed online.

CME INQUIRIES/SPECIAL NEEDS
For all CME inquiries or special needs, please contact elsevierCME@elsevier.com.

SLEEP MEDICINE CLINICS

THE CLINICS ARE AVAILABLE ONLINE!
Access your subscription at:
www.theclinics.com

Contributors

CONSULTING EDITOR

TEOFILO LEE-CHIONG Jr, MD
Professor of Medicine, National Jewish Health;
Professor of Medicine, School of Medicine,
University of Colorado Denver, Denver,
Colorado; Chief Medical Liaison, Philips
Respironics, Pennsylvania

EDITOR

NEIL FREEDMAN, MD
Head, Division of Pulmonary, Critical Care,
Allergy and Immunology, NorthShore
University Health System, Evanston, Illinois

AUTHORS

ROHIT BUDHIRAJA, MD
Division of Pulmonary and Critical Care
Medicine, Department of Medicine; Division of
Sleep and Circadian Disorders, Brigham and
Women's Hospital, Harvard Medical School,
Boston, Massachusetts

PETER C. GAY, MD
Professor of Medicine, Pulmonary, Critical
Care and Sleep Medicine, Mayo Clinic,
Rochester, Minnesota

ROBIN GERMANY, MD
Clinical Assistant Professor of Medicine,
Section of Cardiology, University of Oklahoma
College of Medicine, Oklahoma City,
Oklahoma

ALEX GILELES-HILLEL, MD
Section of Pediatric Sleep Medicine,
Department of Pediatrics, Pritzker School of
Medicine, Biological Sciences Division,
The University of Chicago, Chicago, Illinois

DAVID GOZAL, MD, MBA
Professor, Section of Pediatric Sleep Medicine,
Department of Pediatrics, Pritzker School of
Medicine, Biological Sciences Division,
The University of Chicago, Chicago, Illinois

JOHN J. GREER, PhD
Professor of Physiology, University of Alberta,
Edmonton, Alberta, Canada

DENNIS HWANG, MD
Co-Chair, Sleep Medicine, Southern California
Permanente Medical Group; Medical Director,
Kaiser Permanente Fontana Sleep Disorders
Center, Fontana, California

SHAHROKH JAVAHERI, MD
Sleep Physician, Bethesda North Hospital;
Professor Emeritus of Medicine, University of
Cincinnati College of Medicine, Cincinnati,
Ohio

ABDELNABY KHALYFA, PhD
Associate Professor, Section of Pediatric Sleep
Medicine, Department of Pediatrics, Pritzker
School of Medicine, Biological Sciences
Division, The University of Chicago, Chicago,
Illinois

MATTHEW KIM, MD
Division of Endocrinology, Diabetes and
Hypertension, Department of Medicine,
Brigham and Women's Hospital, Harvard
Medical School, Boston, Massachusetts

TOMASZ J. KUŹNIAR, MD, PhD, FCCP, FAASM
Division of Pulmonary and Critical Care Medicine, NorthShore University HealthSystem, Evanston, Illinois

ATUL MALHOTRA, MD
Professor, Division of Pulmonary and Critical Care Medicine, University of California San Diego, La Jolla, California

TODD D. MORGAN, DMD
Chief, Oral Medicine, Scripps Memorial Hospital, Encinitas, California

ROBERT L. OWENS, MD
Assistant Clinical Professor, Division of Pulmonary and Critical Care Medicine, University of California San Diego, La Jolla, California

SUSAN REDLINE, MD, MPH
Division of Sleep and Circadian Disorders, Brigham and Women's Hospital, Harvard Medical School, Boston, Massachusetts; Division of Pulmonary, Critical Care and Sleep Medicine, Department of Medicine, Beth Israel Deaconess Medical Center, Harvard Medical School, Boston, Massachusetts

SCOTT A. SANDS, PhD
Instructor in Medicine, Division of Sleep and Circadian Disorders, Departments of Medicine and Neurology, Brigham & Women's Hospital and Harvard Medical School, Boston, Massachusetts; Department of Allergy, Immunology and Respiratory Medicine and Central Clinical School, The Alfred and Monash University, Prahran, Victoria, Australia

RONALDO A. SEVILLA BERRIOS, MD
Critical Care Medicine, University of Pittsburg Medical Center at Hamot, Erie, Pennsylvania

RYAN J. SOOSE, MD
Director, UPMC Division of Sleep Surgery; Assistant Professor, Department of Otolaryngology, University of Pittsburgh School of Medicine, Pittsburgh, Pennsylvania

ROBERT THOMAS, MD, MMSc
Division of Pulmonary, Critical Care and Sleep Medicine, Department of Medicine, Beth Israel Deaconess Medical Center, Harvard Medical School, Boston, Massachusetts

DAVID P. WHITE, MD
Professor of Medicine, Part Time, Harvard Medical School, Boston, Massachusetts

Contents

New Approaches to Diagnosing Sleep-Disordered Breathing   143

Scott A. Sands, Robert L. Owens, and Atul Malhotra

> Novel concepts and technological advances have the potential to change the landscape on which clinical sleep medicine is practiced. Screening for sleep apnea will take advantage of readily available mobile telephone technology (sound, accelerometers) to enable widespread recognition of sleep-disordered breathing. Advanced computer-assisted scoring algorithms will improve efficiency and reliability of sleep apnea diagnoses. As the field adopts a personalized approach to therapies, methods to determine the mechanisms of sleep apnea in individuals will be developed—utilizing simplified tests and available recordings—with the promise of predicting outcomes of novel therapies.

New Approaches to Positive Airway Pressure Treatment in Obstructive Sleep Apnea   153

Tomasz J. Kuźniar

> Continuous positive airway pressure (CPAP) is a mainstay of therapy in patients with obstructive sleep apnea (OSA). This technology has gone through tremendous changes that resulted in devices that can recognize and differentiate sleep-disordered breathing events, adjust their output to these events, monitor usage, and communicate with the treatment team. This article discusses recent developments in treatment of OSA with PAP.

Monitoring Progress and Adherence with Positive Airway Pressure Therapy for Obstructive Sleep Apnea: The Roles of Telemedicine and Mobile Health Applications   161

Dennis Hwang

> Technology is changing the way health care is delivered and how patients are approaching their own health. Given the challenge within sleep medicine of optimizing adherence to continuous positive airway pressure (CPAP) therapy in patients with obstructive sleep apnea (OSA), implementation of telemedicine-based mechanisms is a critical component toward developing a comprehensive and cost-effective solution for OSA management. Key elements include the use of electronic messaging, remote monitoring, automated care mechanisms, and patient self-management platforms. Current practical sleep-related telemedicine platforms include Web-based educational programs, automated CPAP follow-up platforms that promote self-management, and peer-based patient-driven Internet support forums.

Novel Approaches to the Management of Sleep-Disordered Breathing   173

Todd D. Morgan

 Video content accompanies this article at http://www.sleep.theclinics.com/

> In the last several years, a variety of novel approaches to the treatment of sleep-disordered breathing have emerged. This new technology holds promise in

serving to re-engage with patients who have previously been lost to follow-up due to continuous positive airway pressure intolerance. With more tools at our disposal, in turn more options can be offered to patients' growing demand for alternatives that are tailored to their individual needs. The key to proper deployment of alternative therapies will often depend on identification of certain phenotypic traits that trend toward a reasonable response to a given therapy.

Novel approaches to upper airway anatomic phenotyping, more reconstructive upper airway surgical techniques, and new implantable hypoglossal neurostimulation technology have very favorable potential to improve symptoms and quality-of-life measures, to reduce obstructive sleep apnea (OSA) disease severity and associated cardiovascular risk, and to serve as an adjunct to continuous positive airway pressure, oral appliances, and other forms of OSA medical therapy. Successful surgical therapy depends critically on accurate diagnosis, skillful knowledge and examination of the upper airway anatomy, proper procedure selection, and proficient technical application.

The concept of pharmacologic therapy for obstructive sleep apnea (OSA) treatment has always been considered, but no agent has had a large enough effect size to drive substantial adoption. A new construct of the pathophysiology of OSA is that there are 4 primary physiologic traits that dictate who develops OSA. These traits vary substantially between patients, meaning OSA may develop for quite different reasons. This encourages new thinking regarding pharmacologic therapy and continued attempts to find the ideal or acceptable drug.

Obstructive sleep apnea (OSA) is a highly prevalent condition that remains underdiagnosed and undertreated. The onerous and labor-intensive nature of polysomnography or similar diagnostic multichannel-based approaches paves the way for exploration of biomarkers aimed at diagnosis, morbidity detection, and monitoring of therapy and its outcomes. To this effect, "Omics" technologies coupled with appropriate bioinformatic approaches should enable discovery of unique biomarker-based signatures, enabling simplified and highly precise algorithms for the evaluation and treatment of symptomatic individuals. Such approaches are likely to not only lead to improved outcomes but also permit personalized medicine to become reality in the context of OSA.

Neurophysiologically, central apnea is due to a temporary cessation of respiratory rhythmogenesis in medullary respiratory networks. Central apneas occur in several disorders and result in pathophysiological consequences, including arousals and desaturation. The 2 most common causes in adults are congestive heart failure and chronic use of opioids to treat pain. Under such circumstances, diagnosis and treatment of central sleep apnea may improve quality of life, morbidity, and mortality. This article discusses recent developments in the treatment of central sleep apnea in heart failure and opioids use.

Analysis of large-volume data holds promise for improving the application of precision medicine to sleep, including improving identification of patient subgroups who may benefit from alternative therapies. Big data used within the health care system also promises to facilitate end-to-end screening, diagnosis, and management of sleep disorders; improve the recognition of differences in presentation and susceptibility to sleep apnea; and lead to improved management and outcomes. To meet the vision of personalized, precision therapeutics and diagnostics and improving the efficiency and quality of sleep medicine will require ongoing efforts, investments, and change in our current medical and research cultures.

Chronic obstructive pulmonary disease (COPD) is a common disease affecting about 20 million US adults. Sleep-disordered breathing (SDB) problems are frequent and poorly characterized for patients with COPD. Both the well-known success of noninvasive ventilation (NIV) in the acute COPD exacerbation in the hospital setting and that NIV is the cornerstone of chronic therapy for SDBs have urged the attention of the medical community to determine the impact of NIV on chronic COPD management with and without coexisting SDBs. Early observational studies showed decreased long-term survival rates on patients with COPD with concomitant chronic hypercapnia when compared with normocapnic patients.

Preface

Novel Approaches to the Management of Sleep-Disordered Breathing: Reviewing the Past and Looking Into the Future

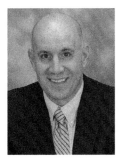

Neil Freedman, MD
Editor

Sleep-disordered breathing means different things to different people. While the term is often used interchangeably with obstructive sleep apnea (OSA), in a broader sense the term refers to the spectrum of breathing disorders that occur, or are exacerbated, during the sleep period. This issue of *Sleep Medicine Clinics*, written by some of the leaders in the field of sleep medicine, reviews many of the recent advancements in the management of sleep-disordered breathing as well as looks into the future of how these disorders will likely be managed.

The majority of the issue is dedicated to the management of OSA. OSA is common, and its prevalence is increasing as our population ages and becomes more overweight. The standard approach to the diagnosis and treatment of OSA involves one or two technician-attended sessions in the sleep lab, typically resulting in the initiation of continuous positive airway pressure (CPAP) therapy. This approach, while comprehensive, is costly and has consistently resulted in CPAP adherence rates of only 50% to 60%. The relatively recent introduction of an out-of-center management approach of OSA with home sleep testing and AutoCPAP has been associated with similar outcomes to the standard approach. While these newer management approaches result in reduced costs, they have not been associated

with improved adherence to therapy or improvements in other important outcomes. Thus, newer approaches to the diagnosis and treatment of OSA are needed.

In this issue, Drs Sands, Owens, and Malhotra initially review the physiology of OSA and examine several current and potential future diagnostic approaches to this disease. The following articles by Drs Kuzniar and Morgan are devoted to advances in the standard OSA treatments, such as CPAP and oral appliance therapies. Dr Hwang reviews how telemedicine and mobile applications may augment and potentially improve how clinicians manage and potentially improve important outcomes with positive airway pressure (PAP) therapy. Surgery can be considered for select groups of patients who are not candidates for, or who cannot tolerate, PAP or oral appliance therapies. In his article, Dr Soose reviews novel surgical approaches to the treatment of OSA. Dr White then reviews current and potential pharmacologic approaches to the treatment of OSA. Finally, two articles are dedicated to reviewing how precision medicine and big data may be used in the future to aid in the management of OSA.

Central sleep apnea (CSA) defines another spectrum of sleep-related breathing disorders characterized by cessations of airflow in the absence of respiratory effort. CSA can be

Sleep Med Clin 11 (2016) xiii–xiv
http://dx.doi.org/10.1016/j.jsmc.2016.03.003
1556-407X/16/$ – see front matter © 2016 Published by Elsevier Inc.

observed in several medical disorders, and a specific type of CSA has been associated with increased morbidity and mortality in patients with congestive heart failure with reduced ejection fraction. Some initial post-hoc analysis data from a large randomized trial demonstrated that CPAP treatment of CSA, in a subgroup of CHF patients, resulted in improved survival and cardiac function. Unfortunately, results from a more recent large randomized trial of adaptive servo ventilation PAP therapy in this patient population demonstrated increased mortality and no improvements in hospitalizations, symptoms, or functional capacity. Thus, newer and better approaches are required to improve outcomes in these patients. Dr Javaheri's article reviews several novel therapies for the management of CSA.

Finally, sleep-related breathing disorders are not limited to OSA and CSA. Chronic obstructive pulmonary disease (COPD) can be associated with several types of sleep-related breathing disorders. Some data suggest that untreated patients with the overlap syndrome (COPD with OSA) have more exacerbations of their chronic lung disease, more hospitalizations, and an overall higher mortality compared with patients with COPD without concomitant OSA. These observational studies also suggest that CPAP treatment can improve many of these outcomes. In addition, there are conflicting data on whether more innovative PAP devices can reduce hospitalizations and improve survival in patients with more advanced lung disease. Drs Berrios and Gay review some of the novel management approaches to patients with COPD and associated sleep-disordered breathing.

As noted previously, we have made many advances in the management of the spectrum of sleep-related breathing disorders. Despite these advances, we still have a long way to go. We need better ways to identify and diagnose at-risk patients and determine the best treatment methods to improve important patient outcomes. This issue of *Sleep Medicine Clinics* should offer the reader some insight into the future of managing these patients and disorders. Enjoy!

Neil Freedman, MD
Division of Pulmonary
Critical Care, Allergy, and Immunology
NorthShore University Health System
2650 Ridge Avenue
Evanston, IL 60201, USA

E-mail address:
nfreedman@northshore.org

New Approaches to Diagnosing Sleep-Disordered Breathing

Scott A. Sands, PhD[a,b,*], Robert L. Owens, MD[c],
Atul Malhotra, MD[c]

KEYWORDS

- Apnea • Screening • Phenotyping • Technology

KEY POINTS

- Home sleep testing is now widely used.
- Advanced analysis of respiratory sounds, electrocardiogram, and body movements will likely enable widespread screening for sleep-disordered breathing.
- Semi-automated scoring algorithms will reduce the resources required and improve consistency of diagnoses.
- Personalized sleep medicine will approach actuality as noninvasive methods reveal sleep apnea mechanisms, allowing clinicians to determine what options are best suited for individual patients.

DETECTING THE PRESENCE OF EVENTS: DIAGNOSTIC AND SCREENING TECHNOLOGY

In-laboratory diagnostic polysomnography has traditionally been the gold standard for obstructive sleep apnea (OSA) diagnosis, but the high prevalence of disease and the massive number of patients at risk of disease cannot reasonably be diagnosed at in-laboratory facilities. Peppard and colleagues[1] conservatively estimated that 10% of the US population has clinically important OSA, suggesting more than 30 million people afflicted with OSA in the United States alone. Clearly, many more are at risk of OSA or have more mild disease. Heinzer and colleagues[2] used gold-standard techniques in Switzerland and estimated up to 50% of men had some degree of clinically important apnea. Thus, the use of new technology to detect respiratory events (without the need for cumbersome and expensive in-laboratory testing) is an important step forward. Home sleep testing (HST) provides acceptable diagnostic sensitivity and specificity, although most technologies cannot distinguish wake from sleep, non-rapid eye movement (NREM) from rapid eye movement (REM) sleep, or supine from lateral posture. As a result, clinicians get only partial information when determining therapy.

Disclosures: Dr S.A. Sands was supported by the National Health and Medical Research Council of Australia and the R.G. Menzies Foundation (1053201, 1035115) and is currently supported by the American Heart Association (15SDG25890059). Dr R.L. Owens consults for Apnex Medical, Apnicure, and Philips Respironics. Dr A. Malhotra was a consultant for Philips Respironics, SHC, SGS, Apnex Medical, Pfizer, and Apnicure, but has relinquished all outside personal income since May 2012.
[a] Division of Sleep and Circadian Disorders, Departments of Medicine and Neurology, Brigham & Women's Hospital and Harvard Medical School, 221 Longwood Avenue, Boston, MA 02115, USA; [b] Department of Allergy, Immunology and Respiratory Medicine and Central Clinical School, The Alfred and Monash University, 55 Commercial Road, Prahran, Victoria 3181, Australia; [c] Division of Pulmonary and Critical Care Medicine, University of California San Diego, 9500 Gilman Dr La Jolla, CA 92093, USA
* Corresponding author. Division of Sleep and Circadian Disorders, Departments of Medicine and Neurology, Brigham & Women's Hospital and Harvard Medical School, Boston, MA.
E-mail address: sasands@partners.org

Sleep Med Clin 11 (2016) 143–152
http://dx.doi.org/10.1016/j.jsmc.2016.01.005

sleep.theclinics.com

Home Sleep Testing

HST has been used widely around the world and has recently increased in popularity in the United States. The factors driving home testing are primarily financial given the realization of the massive numbers of patients who may need to undergo testing and the data suggesting a satisfactory clinical result can be obtained using a HST approach. Several randomized trials were completed that compared the results of HST plus in home auto-titration positive airway pressure (PAP) therapy versus usual care via in-laboratory polysomnography or split night testing.[3-9] Although still the topic of debate,[10,11] the data in aggregate support a home testing approach suggesting equal if not better outcomes using home testing as compared with the traditional approach. An important caveat, however, is that most studies have carefully screened for patients at risk for moderate to severe OSA and studied patients without comorbid medical disorders (eg, chronic obstructive pulmonary disease, heart failure, obesity-hypoventilation, opioids for chronic pain).

A variety of devices are available for HST, each with potential strengths and weaknesses. In general, simple equipment provides fewer channels and potentially less data to interpret, whereas more complex equipment can record multiple channels but can be more cumbersome to use and interpret. The authors think that the number of channels on a given device is less relevant than the sensitivity and specificity of the device and the clinical outcomes that a given device can achieve. Thus, the classification system based on number of channels, for example, level 2 versus level 3, is not particularly helpful.

Given the appropriate reliance on home testing, many subtleties are worth mentioning:

a. Given that home testing rarely monitors body position in a robust manner, positional therapy becomes hard to implement in the HST era. Positional therapy can be useful for patients who are intolerant of continuous positive airway pressure (CPAP) or as an adjunctive therapy in patients with partial response to therapies such as weight loss or oral appliance therapy. Thus, in-laboratory testing or other methods of position monitoring may have a role for select patients.

b. Respiratory events may have varying impact depending on whether they occur during REM sleep versus NREM sleep. Because REM sleep is characterized by physiologic variability, some have argued that respiratory fluctuations during REM sleep may not have major consequences. On the other hand, some recent data do support clinically important impact of respiratory events during REM sleep.[12,13] Moreover, some patients experience profound desaturations during REM sleep, presumably as a result of skeletal muscle atonia in accessory respiratory muscles. These profound desaturations are unlikely to be physiologic and thus likely require therapy. As a result, CPAP therapy is often prescribed for both REM and NREM events, making the distinction during diagnostic testing between these 2 states less important clinically.

c. Because most HST devices do not monitor sleep, the devices work on the assumption that the total recording time is actually the total sleep time, that is, that the patient sleeps 100% of the night. As a result, the apnea hypopnea index (AHI) as judged by HST can underestimate the actual AHI, particularly among patients with reduced sleep efficiency. For example, a patient with 50% sleep efficiency who has an AHI of 4/h may actually have an AHI = 8/h if the impact of poor sleep quality was addressed. Thus, the interpretation of HST must be made cautiously in patients with comorbid insomnia or in patients who report poor sleep quality during the recording.

d. When sleep is not monitored, the HST-reported AHI may underestimate hypopneas that terminate as arousals from sleep. In particular, younger and leaner patients who have normal cardiopulmonary function (ie, normal lung volume, alveolar-arterial gradient), and thus less prone to oxygen desaturation for any given reduction in airflow, may not exhibit frequent (eg, >3%) desaturation events but may still have sleep fragmentation. These events may not meet criteria because arousals cannot be scored on most home devices. Home devices that do assess sleep stages and arousals may thus have additional value over those that ignore sleep staging.

Novel Approaches to Screening and Monitoring Sleep Apnea

For the large-scale screening for sleep apnea, even the most accurate HST is limited because of the availability of equipment. For longer-term monitoring of sleep apnea, in the era of patient-directed health management, the requirement for sensors to be placed on the body is an additional limitation. Novel screening approaches typically do not measure directly the key features of sleep apnea (airflow, oxygen levels, electroencephalogram [EEG] arousal) but instead rely on surrogate measurements with a reduction in accuracy as a tradeoff for broader applicability.

Snoring and breathing sounds

Many patients with OSA present initially with witnessed abnormal breathing sounds such as snoring and gasping at night. On the basis that OSA is audible, researchers suspect that sleep apnea might be identifiable by listening to at-risk patients breathe during sleep. Evidence to date suggests that indeed sleep apnea may be distinguished from nonapneic snoring by variations in snoring sound intensity with cyclic apneas and hypopneas. Harnessing this information with the recording and advanced analysis of respiratory sounds is arguably the most promising approach to large-scale screening for sleep apnea. Given the broad availability of mobile telephone devices with sufficient computational power and microphones, the current challenge lies in the development, implementation, and validation of robust tools to screen for sleep apnea that are applicable in the home and effective across device platforms. Although no such validated approach currently exists, investigators are enthusiastically developing this technology.

A popular approach has been to examine several candidate features of snoring/respiratory sounds across the night and use these in statistical models to select the most useful features to predict (yes or no) whether a patient has sleep apnea (based on concurrent gold-standard polysomnography recordings).[14] A potential limitation of this approach is that apneas/hypopneas are not identified on an event-by-event basis, but by global features that correlate with OSA. A more powerful approach may be to identify which features specifically relate to individual respiratory events. In this context, a relatively simple approach to event detection, used by Nakano and colleagues,[15] made use of the concept that apneas/hypopneas are generally accompanied by relative dips and surges in sound power. Using a mobile smartphone placed on the chest, the frequency of 3-dB dips in time-averaged sound power (50–2000 Hz, 20-second averaging time) were counted and compared with the frequency of OSA events, yielding a relatively accurate means to screen patients for sleep apnea (r = 0.94, receiver operating characteristic area = 0.92). Importantly, this accuracy was achieved in a sleep laboratory, without the influence of sounds from a bed partner or the home environment. Although the challenges of unsupervised use outside the laboratory setting have not yet been overcome,

the use of snoring sounds as a screening tool has tremendous potential. Central apneas are likely to represent a separate challenge because their sound characteristics are presumably quite different from those of OSA. Future methods may use multiple sound features to identify individual respiratory events more accurately.

Electrocardiogram

The recording of electrocardiograms (EKG) via Holter monitors or implantable cardiac devices is used extensively in the diagnosis and monitoring of cardiovascular diseases. Given that sleep apnea promotes cardiovascular disease, and vice versa, screening for sleep apnea in this at-risk population is of major interest. Fifteen years ago, Physionet and Computers in Cardiology proposed a challenge to the field to develop techniques to detect sleep apnea on an epoch-by-epoch basis, and to classify individuals as apneic or nonapneic using EKG alone.[16] The resulting methods, and those developed thereafter, have illustrated that the EKG provides a rich source of information for the identification of individuals with likely sleep apnea.

The EKG signal varies with respiration in 2 primary ways. Tidal respiration increases lung volume and the increased thoracic gas volume, thereby raising the thoracic electrical impedance, and in turn, reducing the amplitude of the EKG signal; alterations in the axis of the heart relative to the electrodes may play a further role. Thus, tracking the amplitude of the QRS complex across breaths (EKG-derived respiration) provides a means to observe the cyclic changes in tidal volume that characterize sleep apnea.[17] Heart rate also varies in a cyclic manner in concert with the sleep apnea cycle and provides additional information that can be used for sleep apnea screening[18,19]; day-night differences in heart rate variability may also be of utility.[20] Combined fluctuations in heart rate and EKG amplitude can yield surprisingly accurate classification of sleep apnea.[17,19,21,22] Further research is required, however, because it remains uncertain whether the available methods have utility across patients with a variety of cardiovascular comorbidities and accompanying differences in cardiac rhythm (eg, ectopic beats), heart rate variability, or the presence of paced beats (eg, in heart failure).[23]

Motion detection

The use of accelerometers to quantify motion has become widespread in the last decade across multiple fields. Since the 1990s, motion detection in the form of an actigraph worn most commonly on the wrist has been used to assess rest periods (presumed sleep) in the field of sleep.[24] For the purpose of sleep apnea diagnosis, however, actigraph determination of sleep duration may not provide much additional accuracy when coupled with HST devices (number of events per hour of sleep),[25,26] possibly given difficulties detecting arousals or wakefulness within an extended sleep period.[27] Nevertheless, motion detection may be applied to assess the dynamic respiratory movements and screen for sleep-disordered breathing.[28,29]

AUTOMATED AND COMPUTER-ASSISTED SCORING TECHNOLOGY

Sleep technicians have generally scored in-laboratory polysomnographic recordings manually. With the move toward home testing, there is less of a need for sleep technicians to perform manual scoring of sleep. Home testing devices have automated algorithms in some cases that are reasonably accurate, although review of raw data can often be revealing in the context of artifacts. Efforts to make in-laboratory polysomnography more useful have included attempts to garner more information than just the AHI and have involved efforts to automate or partially automate scoring of the data.

The automated versus manual approaches have associated risks and benefits. Proponents of the automated approach cite data regarding reproducibility of computer algorithms versus human judgment. In addition, human fatigue during scoring is not an issue with automated approaches. Moreover, automated systems can be considerably faster and cheaper than human technicians, allowing scalable approaches to be applied to large numbers of patients. Proponents of manual approaches point to the existing gold standards, which have been used to develop current guidelines. In addition, human experience can be valuable because artifacts that can be identified easily by inspection may "fool" computer algorithms if not adequately trained. Some have also argued that loss of employment for sleep technicians may have a major detrimental effect on the field, even though their efforts could perhaps be redirected to assisting with follow-up and PAP adherence. As the automated algorithms improve, they are being gradually adopted clinically, although the utility of human judgment and experience is still valued. Thus, semi-automated or computer-assisted techniques for scoring sleep studies are likely to become the standard in the future.

Sleep State and Arousals

Computational measurement of EEG has long been used to stage sleep and detect arousals. Most commonly, methods have used EEG spectral analysis. Here two papers are briefly highlighted. In a small number of participants, Asyali and colleagues[30] demonstrated that arousals from sleep could be detected automatically using absolute beta power (16–25 Hz), an EEG frequency range that was preferable in comparison to lower frequency bands (delta, theta, alpha). Recently, Younes and colleagues[31] quantified EEG power in 3-second epochs and assigned each epoch 4 values based on the delta, theta, alpha, and beta powers (in deciles). For each combination of EEG power deciles (from [0, 0, 0, 0] to [9, 9, 9, 9], lookup tables are proprietary, not provided), the likelihood of occurring during technician-scored wake was calculated. These values have been validated to predict sleep or wake with high accuracy versus traditional 30-second technician-scored epochs. The method has been incorporated into a system to both stage polysomnographic studies and score respiratory events.[32] A potential weakness of both approaches is the reliance on absolute EEG power, such that a smaller amplitude signal, for example, due to electrical properties of the scalp or lead impedances, will reduce the EEG power in all bands and thereby affect the estimated sleep stage. The authors expect further development of proprietary and publicly available techniques to robustly quantify sleep using computational analysis of the EEG in the coming years.

Respiratory Events

Compared with the detection of sleep stage, automated assessment of respiratory events appears relatively straightforward. However, several major impediments remain. First, apneas and hypopneas are defined typically as a 30% and 90% reduction in airflow from a preceding baseline level (noting that signal amplitude may drift overnight if airflow sensors are not maintained precisely in place). Nevertheless, during cyclic breathing, there is no clear baseline level. Thus, manual scorers and automated systems will vary simply because of the use of different definitions of baseline respiration. Novel approaches are needed to ascertain what baseline eupneic ventilation is (eg, the ventilation that maintains normal arterial blood gases). Second, respiratory events are usually assessed using nasal pressure rather than true airflow via a pneumotachograph and full face mask (or nasal mask with the mouth confirmed to be closed). Nasal pressure (Pnasal) is related to true ventilation (Vflow) via an approximately square relationship (Pnasal $\approx$ k.Vflow^2) with different coefficients for inspiration and expiration.[33]

Some systems use a square-root transform of nasal pressure to approximately linearize the signal to better relate to the relative changes in Vflow. This approach, however, may overestimate the flow signal at small amplitudes such that further improvement is warranted. Third, the classification of apneas and hypopneas as either obstructive (flow is reduced due primarily to upper airway narrowing) or central (due to reduced neural drive) remains a major challenge. In the absence of measures of diaphragm electromyogram or esophageal/epiglottic pressure, manual scorers rely on nuances in nasal pressure flow morphology (flattening, scooping, flutter, increase in inspiratory time), or phase shifts or paradox seen between the thoracic and abdominal belts, to determine whether a hypopnea is obstructive rather than central. Automation of these methods is still in its infancy.[34]

APPROACHES TO DIAGNOSING SLEEP APNEA PATHOPHYSIOLOGY FOR GUIDING TREATMENT DECISIONS

Personalized medicine has become a major source of discussion for many diseases, including OSA. Recent evidence has supported the notion that many mechanisms underlie OSA and that identification of these underlying endotypes can help to individualize therapy for a given individual. OSA is now recognized to be a disease of anatomic compromise with variable underlying pathophysiological mechanisms, including compromised upper airway dilator muscle activity, unstable ventilatory control (elevated loop gain), and low arousal threshold, among others. At least in theory, therapies to address these underlying mechanisms may be particularly effective in resolving apnea. Some patients may have multiple underlying mechanisms, in which case combination therapies would be predicted to eliminate apnea. For example, patients that compromise primarily at the level of the velopharynx would be predicted to respond well to uvulopalatopharyngoplasty. Similarly, patients with dysfunction in the upper airway dilator muscles may be particularly good candidates for hypoglossal nerve stimulation. Currently, OSA diagnostics yield only an AHI as an imperfect measure of sleep apnea severity but make little attempt to provide pathophysiological insight.

Here the literature knowledge is summarized, relating 4 key pathophysiological phenotypes of sleep apnea to the clinical manifestation of this disease. Overall, there is considerable evidence that pathophysiological phenotypes manifest clinically in recognizable ways. Novel methods to noninvasively quantify these phenotypes are needed to enable judicious matching of patients to emerging therapies.

Upper Airway Collapsibility: Severity

The gold-standard functional assessment of upper airway collapsibility is the critical collapsing pressure (Pcrit) measured in the anesthetized state, or during sleep when the upper airway dilator muscles are minimally active. Pcrit is defined as the level of nasal (upstream) pressure at which the upper airway collapses and is the X-intercept of a peak-flow versus nasal pressure plot. Alternatively, collapsibility can be assessed by calculating the Y-intercept of such a plot, providing the level of peak flow (or ventilation, Vpassive) at atmospheric pressure under maximally passive conditions.

Several investigators have attempted to estimate collapsibility using simpler and more clinically relevant measures, generally during wakefulness. These measures include, but are not limited to, measures of body habitus (neck circumference, body mass index), visual assessment of the upper airway (Mallampati/Friedman scores), and measures of patency/collapsibility during wakefulness (acoustic pharyngometry,[35] negative pressure pulses during expiration[36]).

The potential utility of several polysomnographic indicators of a more collapsible *passive* upper airway are highlighted:

- In comparison to NREM sleep, upper airway dilator muscles are less active during REM sleep.[37] The severity of REM sleep apnea (AHI) is more closely related to passive collapsibility than the severity of sleep apnea during NREM.[38–40] Likewise, at the other end of the spectrum, patients with primarily central sleep apnea (and presumably minimal collapsibility) typically exhibit a low AHI in REM. REM AHI may therefore be a marker of passive collapsibility.
- A greater therapeutic CPAP requirement is also expected to indicate a more collapsible upper airway. On CPAP, upper airway muscle activity is minimal. The therapeutic CPAP therefore reflects the level that slightly exceeds the value on the passive pressure flow curve that yields flow limitation.
- Patients whose sleep apnea resolves with lateral positioning (supine predominant) have a less collapsible upper airway than those with sleep apnea in both the supine and the lateral positions.[41] Indeed, supine predominance, as an indicator of milder collapsibility, is modestly predictive of successful oral appliance therapy.

A severely compromised passive collapsibility has been found previously to explain the failures of nonanatomical therapies targeting loop gain.[42]

Upper Airway Muscle Compensation

During sleep, increased upper airway resistance leads to an increase in ventilatory drive, which stimulates the upper airway dilator muscles to respond. In some individuals, these muscles effectively yield collapsibility (*active* collapsibility vs passive collapsibility) seen as an improvement in ventilation. The active collapsibility is actually a complex variable that is determined not only by the passive collapsibility but also by (1) the increase in muscle activity for a given increase in neural ventilatory drive (muscle responsiveness); (2) the ability of muscle activity to stiffen the airway and improve ventilation; and finally, (3) the ventilatory drive stimulus that can be provided without arousal from sleep (arousal threshold). Also, if the airway is not maximally activated (ie, just before arousal), the measurement may also be affected by loop gain (higher loop gain will yield more drive and thus more activation for any given drop in airflow).

Putative measures of active collapsibility or muscle compensation include the following:

- Apneas versus hypopneas. Compared with patients exhibiting hypopneas, those who consistently exhibit apneas (zero airflow at atmospheric pressure), even when the upper airway dilator muscles are maximally activated (just before arousal), by definition, have a severely compromised active collapsibility (active Pcrit >0).[43] The relative proportion of obstructive apneas versus obstructive hypopneas may therefore reflect the active collapsibility.
- REM predominant sleep apnea, where sleep apnea is more severe in REM versus NREM, is likely to be an indicator of effective upper airway compensation.[40]
- Rather than an a compensatory improvement in ventilation, some individuals exhibit a paradoxic reduction in airflow when ventilatory drive is increased, presumably a combined result of insufficient dilator muscle activation and a highly compliant upper airway. This behavior is referred to as *negative effort dependence*[44–47] (more effort yields less airflow), and this tendency may be detected within-breaths as a substantial reduction in airflow at mid-inspiration versus the peak flow. Therapies that increase ventilatory drive (eg, acetazolamide) are likely to be coundereffective in this patient subgroup.

Evidence for the predictive utility of active collapsibility includes the recent finding that a greater active anatomy is a strong predictor of the response to nonanatomical therapy (loop gain, arousal threshold).[48] In principle, increasing the arousal threshold will have a maximally beneficial effect when the upper airway muscles are effective. Reducing loop gain will also have maximal utility in patients that are able to sustain a reasonable level of airflow.

Upper Airway Collapsibility: Site

Alongside the severity of pharyngeal collapse, there is an increasing awareness of the heterogeneity of the sites and structures involved. These structures include the velum or soft palate, the lateral walls, the base of the tongue, and the epiglottis.

Evidence is accumulating that the site of collapse is important for determining the effectiveness of non-CPAP anatomic therapies. Based on gold-standard upper airway visualization, available data indicate that oral appliances work most effectively in patients with tongue-base collapse,[49] but not those with isolated velum or epiglottic collapse.[50,51] Patients with isolated velum collapse may have better outcomes following uvulopalatopharyngoplasty.

Here 2 noninvasive approaches to detecting the site of collapse are highlighted. First, snoring sound analysis has been used to distinguish between velum and tongue-base collapse. Velum involvement exhibits a characteristic large-amplitude, low-frequency, narrow-band fluttering, whereas tongue-based collapse yields a high-frequency broad-band signal.[52,53] Second, the intrabreath flow shape may also consist of useful information on the site of collapse. For example, patients whose inspiratory flow pattern appears as a simple flat-top (Starling resistor) tend to exhibit tongue-base collapse (a larger, noncompliant structure), whereas those with a substantial reduction from peak flow to midinspiratory flow (degree of *negative effort dependence*) tend to exhibit collapse of highly compliant structures (velum, lateral wall, or epiglottis).[54]

High Loop Gain

Beyond upper airway physiology, a key trait causing sleep apnea is the sensitivity and stability of the ventilatory control system, a feedback loop that acts to maintain ventilation and arterial blood gases near an equilibrium. This sensitivity/stability is typically quantified by the loop gain, which reflects the increase in ventilatory drive that occurs due to a reduction in ventilation. In the absence of a collapsible upper airway, an excessive loop gain results in central sleep apnea. However, increasing loop gain can cause OSA in those with a collapsible airway.[55–58]

The authors recently developed a method to measure loop gain from the overshoot-undershoot ventilatory pattern observed in routine polysomnography. In essence, the method fits a simplified ventilatory control system model to the available data. For any given patient, the best model is that which most accurately converts the reduction in ventilation during apneas/hypopneas to the observed ventilatory drive overshoot seen after each apnea/hypopnea. The method showed a promising ability to detect a high loop gain and predict responses to oxygen and acetazolamide.[59] Further work is needed to (1) more accurately define baseline ventilation, flow-limited breathing, and effects of arousals on ventilatory drive; (2) validate estimated ventilatory drive with respect to gold-standard drive measured with diaphragm muscle activity; and (3) to extend the approach to estimate the remaining traits.

There are several additional indicators of a high loop gain:

- The presence of central or mixed events[60]
- Shorter events and faster cycling between events[59]
- NREM dominant sleep apnea (NREM AHI > REM AHI)
- Relative hypocapnia[61]

In patients with central sleep apnea, the duration of central apneas as a fraction of the cycle period (time from the start of one event to the next) is a direct reflection of the underlying loop gain.[62] This approach has been used to detect those with extremely high loop gain and predict the acute failure of CPAP in patients with heart failure,[62] and the persistence of central events despite 4 weeks of therapy in OSA patients with complex sleep apnea.[63]

Arousal Threshold, Sleep State Instability

Most patients, even those with severe sleep apnea, exhibit stable breathing for some period of the night. Stable breathing often occurs in slow-wave sleep, likely due in part to an increase in the ventilatory drive that can be tolerated before arousal (increased arousal threshold compared with stage N2). In fact, there is a subset of patients with a low arousal threshold or sleep instability, whose sleep apnea may be ameliorated with hypnotics/sedatives to increase the arousal threshold.[64] In principle, raising the arousal threshold has 2 effects on sleep apnea

physiology: (1) it allows a lower level of ventilation (eg, more severe collapsibility) to be tolerated, and (2) it allows a greater level of ventilatory drive to build up, providing a greater stimulus for upper airway muscle activation.[56,65] It is also likely that this treatment approach will be most successful in those with a relatively good active collapsibility. Drugs that promote slow-wave sleep may also be advantageous in these patients.

The authors recently developed a clinical score to identify patients with a low arousal threshold, which incorporates just 3 readily available parameters. One point is given for each of nadir saturation greater than 82.5%, the fraction of hypopneas (vs total respiratory events) greater than 58.3%, and AHI less than 30 events per hour; a score of 2 or greater correctly predicted a low- or high-arousal threshold in 84% of patients.[66] Further investigation is needed to test whether this approach helps to explain responses to therapies that increase the arousal threshold and stabilize sleep in patients with sleep apnea.

SUMMARY

A host of new ideas and advances in technology has the potential to reshape the way clinical sleep medicine is practiced. Advances in analysis of respiratory sounds and EKG will likely enable widespread screening for sleep-disordered breathing. The use of automated scoring algorithms seeks to improve the resources required and consistency of diagnoses. Personalized medicine is one step closer: methods are rapidly being developed to determine the mechanisms of sleep apnea and determine what options are best suited for individual patients.

REFERENCES

1. Peppard PE, Young T, Barnet JH, et al. Increased prevalence of sleep-disordered breathing in adults. Am J Epidemiol 2013;177(9):1006–14.
2. Heinzer R, Vat S, Marques-Vidal P, et al. Prevalence of sleep-disordered breathing in the general population: the HypnoLaus study. Lancet Respir Med 2015; 3:310–8.
3. Mulgrew AT, Fox N, Ayas NT, et al. Diagnosis and initial management of obstructive sleep apnea without polysomnography: a randomized validation study. Ann Intern Med 2007;146:157–66.
4. Chai-Coetzer CL, Antic NA, Rowland LS, et al. Primary care vs specialist sleep center management of obstructive sleep apnea and daytime sleepiness and quality of life: a randomized trial. JAMA 2013; 309:997–1004.
5. Rosen CL, Auckley D, Benca R, et al. A multisite randomized trial of portable sleep studies and

positive airway pressure autotitration versus laboratory-based polysomnography for the diagnosis and treatment of obstructive sleep apnea: the HomePAP study. Sleep 2012;35:757–67.

6. Kuna ST, Gurubhagavatula I, Maislin G, et al. Noninferiority of functional outcome in ambulatory management of obstructive sleep apnea. Am J Respir Crit Care Med 2011;183:1238–44.

7. Skomro RP, Gjevre J, Reid J, et al. Outcomes of home-based diagnosis and treatment of obstructive sleep apnea. Chest 2010;138:257–63.

8. Antic NA, Buchan C, Esterman A, et al. A randomized controlled trial of nurse-led care for symptomatic moderate-severe obstructive sleep apnea. Am J Respir Crit Care Med 2009;179:501–8.

9. Berry RB, Hill G, Thompson L, et al. Portable monitoring and autotitration versus polysomnography for the diagnosis and treatment of sleep apnea. Sleep 2008;31:1423–31.

10. Freedman N. COUNTERPOINT: does laboratory polysomnography yield better outcomes than home sleep testing? No. Chest 2015;148:308–10.

11. Pack AI. POINT: does laboratory polysomnography yield better outcomes than home sleep testing? Yes. Chest 2015;148:306–8.

12. Mokhlesi B, Finn LA, Hagen EW, et al. Obstructive sleep apnea during REM sleep and hypertension. Results of the Wisconsin Sleep Cohort. Am J Respir Crit Care Med 2014;190:1158–67.

13. Mokhlesi B, Hagen EW, Finn LA, et al. Obstructive sleep apnoea during REM sleep and incident non-dipping of nocturnal blood pressure: a longitudinal analysis of the Wisconsin Sleep Cohort. Thorax 2015;70(11):1062–9.

14. Ben-Israel N, Tarasiuk A, Zigel Y. Obstructive apnea hypopnea index estimation by analysis of nocturnal snoring signals in adults. Sleep 2012;35:1299–1305C.

15. Nakano H, Hirayama K, Sadamitsu Y, et al. Monitoring sound to quantify snoring and sleep apnea severity using a smartphone: proof of concept. J Clin Sleep Med 2014;10:73–8.

16. Penzel T, McNames J, Murray A, et al. Systematic comparison of different algorithms for apnoea detection based on electrocardiogram recordings. Med Biol Eng Comput 2002;40:402–7.

17. Babaeizadeh S, Zhou SH, Pittman SD, et al. Electrocardiogram-derived respiration in screening of sleep-disordered breathing. J Electrocardiol 2011;44:700–6.

18. Stein PK, Duntley SP, Domitrovich PP, et al. A simple method to identify sleep apnea using Holter recordings. J Cardiovasc Electrophysiol 2003;14:467–73.

19. Varon C, Caicedo A, Testelmans D, et al. A novel algorithm for the automatic detection of sleep apnea from single-lead ECG. IEEE Trans Biomed Eng 2015;62:2269–78.

20. Roche F, Gaspoz JM, Court-Fortune I, et al. Screening of obstructive sleep apnea syndrome by heart rate variability analysis. Circulation 1999;100:1411–5.

21. de Chazal P, Heneghan C, Sheridan E, et al. Automated processing of the single-lead electrocardiogram for the detection of obstructive sleep apnoea. IEEE Trans Biomed Eng 2003;50:686–96.

22. Heneghan C, de Chazal P, Ryan S, et al. Electrocardiogram recording as a screening tool for sleep disordered breathing. J Clin Sleep Med 2008;4:223–8.

23. Damy T, D'Ortho MP, Estrugo B, et al. Heart rate increment analysis is not effective for sleep-disordered breathing screening in patients with chronic heart failure. J Sleep Res 2010;19:131–8.

24. Martin JL, Hakim AD. Wrist actigraphy. Chest 2011;139:1514–27.

25. Elbaz M, Roue GM, Lofaso F, et al. Utility of actigraphy in the diagnosis of obstructive sleep apnea. Sleep 2002;25:527–31.

26. Garcia-Diaz E, Quintana-Gallego E, Ruiz A, et al. Respiratory polygraphy with actigraphy in the diagnosis of sleep apnea-hypopnea syndrome. Chest 2007;131:725–32.

27. Fonseca P, Long X, Foussier J, et al. On the impact of arousals on the performance of sleep and wake classification using actigraphy. Conf Proc IEEE Eng Med Biol Soc 2013;2013:6760–3.

28. Paalasmaa J, Leppakorpi L, Partinen M. Quantifying respiratory variation with force sensor measurements. Conf Proc IEEE Eng Med Biol Soc 2011;2011:3812–5.

29. Norman MB, Middleton S, Erskine O, et al. Validation of the Sonomat: a contactless monitoring system used for the diagnosis of sleep disordered breathing. Sleep 2014;37:1477–87.

30. Asyali MH, Berry RB, Khoo MC, et al. Determining a continuous marker for sleep depth. Comput Biol Med 2007;37:1600–9.

31. Younes M, Ostrowski M, Soiferman M, et al. Odds ratio product of sleep EEG as a continuous measure of sleep state. Sleep 2015;38:641–54.

32. Malhotra A, Younes M, Kuna ST, et al. Performance of an automated polysomnography scoring system versus computer-assisted manual scoring. Sleep 2013;36:573–82.

33. Montserrat JM, Farre R, Ballester E, et al. Evaluation of nasal prongs for estimating nasal flow. Am J Respir Crit Care Med 1997;155:211–5.

34. Mooney AM, Abounasr KK, Rapoport DM, et al. Relative prolongation of inspiratory time predicts high versus low resistance categorization of hypopneas. J Clin Sleep Med 2012;8:177–85.

35. Deyoung PN, Bakker JP, Sands SA, et al. Acoustic pharyngometry measurement of minimal cross-sectional airway area is a significant independent

predictor of moderate-to-severe obstructive sleep apnea. J Clin Sleep Med 2013;9:1161–4.

36. Montemurro LT, Bettinzoli M, Corda L, et al. Relationship between critical pressure and volume exhaled during negative pressure in awake subjects with sleep-disordered breathing. Chest 2010;137: 1304–9.

37. Eckert DJ, Malhotra A, Lo YL, et al. The influence of obstructive sleep apnea and gender on genioglossus activity during rapid eye movement sleep. Chest 2009;135:957–64.

38. Eastwood PR, Szollosi I, Platt PR, et al. Comparison of upper airway collapse during general anaesthesia and sleep. Lancet 2002;359:1207–9.

39. Chin CH, Kirkness JP, Patil SP, et al. Compensatory responses to upper airway obstruction in obese apneic men and women. J Appl Physiol (1985) 2012;112:403–10.

40. Sands SA, Eckert DJ, Jordan AS, et al. Enhanced upper-airway muscle responsiveness is a distinct feature of overweight/obese individuals without sleep apnea. Am J Respir Crit Care Med 2014; 190(8):930–7.

41. Joosten SA, Edwards BA, Wellman A, et al. The effect of body position on physiological factors that contribute to obstructive sleep apnea. Sleep 2015; 38(9):1469–78.

42. Xie A, Teodorescu M, Pegelow DF, et al. Effects of stabilizing or increasing respiratory motor outputs on obstructive sleep apnea. J Appl Physiol (1985) 2013;115(1):22–33.

43. Gleadhill IC, Schwartz AR, Schubert N, et al. Upper airway collapsibility in snorers and in patients with obstructive hypopnea and apnea. Am Rev Respir Dis 1991;143:1300–3.

44. Owens RL, Edwards BA, Sands SA, et al. Upper airway collapsibility and patterns of flow limitation at constant end-expiratory lung volume. J Appl Physiol (1985) 2012;113:691–9.

45. Owens RL, Edwards BA, Sands SA, et al. The classical Starling resistor model often does not predict inspiratory airflow patterns in the human upper airway. J Appl Physiol (1985) 2014;116:1105–12.

46. Genta PR, Owens RL, Edwards BA, et al. Influence of pharyngeal muscle activity on inspiratory negative effort dependence in the human upper airway. Respir Physiol Neurobiol 2014;201:55–9.

47. Wellman A, Genta PR, Owens RL, et al. Test of the Starling resistor model in the human upper airway during sleep. J Appl Physiol (1985) 2014;117: 1478–85.

48. Edwards BA, Sands SA, Owens RL, et al. Combination therapy for the treatment of obstructive sleep apnea [abstract]. Am J Respir Crit Care Med 2013; 187:A3759.

49. Ng AT, Qian J, Cistulli PA. Oropharyngeal collapse predicts treatment response with oral appliance therapy in obstructive sleep apnea. Sleep 2006;29: 666–71.

50. Vanderveken OM, Dieltjens M, Wouters K, et al. Drug-induced Sedation Endoscopy (DISE) findings correlate with treatment outcome in OSA patients treated with oral appliance therapy in a fixed mandibular protrusion [abstract]. Am J Respir Crit Care Med 2015;191:A2474.

51. Vanderveken OM, Maurer JT, Hohenhorst W, et al. Evaluation of drug-induced sleep endoscopy as a patient selection tool for implanted upper airway stimulation for obstructive sleep apnea. J Clin Sleep Med 2013;9:433–8.

52. Osborne JE, Osman EZ, Hill PD, et al. A new acoustic method of differentiating palatal from non-palatal snoring. Clin Otolaryngol allied Sci 1999;24:130–3.

53. Agrawal S, Stone P, McGuinness K, et al. Sound frequency analysis and the site of snoring in natural and induced sleep. Clin Otolaryngol allied Sci 2002;27:162–6.

54. Genta PR, Edwards BA, Sands SA, et al. Identifying the upper airway structure causing collapse in obstructive sleep apnea by the shape of airflow [abstract]. Am J Respir Crit Care Med 2015;191: A5604.

55. Wellman A, Jordan AS, Malhotra A, et al. Ventilatory control and airway anatomy in obstructive sleep apnea. Am J Respir Crit Care Med 2004;170: 1225–32.

56. Wellman A, Edwards BA, Sands SA, et al. A simplified method for determining phenotypic traits in patients with obstructive sleep apnea. J Appl Physiol 2013;114:911–22.

57. Eckert DJ, White DP, Jordan AS, et al. Defining phenotypic causes of obstructive sleep apnea. Identification of novel therapeutic targets. Am J Respir Crit Care Med 2013;188:996–1004.

58. Edwards BA, Sands SA, Eckert DJ, et al. Acetazolamide improves loop gain but not the other physiological traits causing obstructive sleep apnoea. J Physiol 2012;590:1199–211.

59. Terrill P, Edwards BA, Nemati S, et al. Quantifying the ventilatory control contribution to sleep apnea using polysomnography. Eur Respir J 2015;45(2): 408–18.

60. Xie A, Bedekar A, Skatrud JB, et al. The heterogeneity of obstructive sleep apnea (predominant obstructive vs pure obstructive apnea). Sleep 2011;34:745–50.

61. Xie A, Rutherford R, Rankin F, et al. Hypocapnia and increased ventilatory responsiveness in patients with idiopathic central sleep apnea. Am J Respir Crit Care Med 1995;152:1950–5.

62. Sands SA, Edwards BA, Kee K, et al. Loop gain as a means to predict a positive airway pressure suppression of Cheyne-Stokes respiration in patients

with heart failure. Am J Respir Crit Care Med 2011; 184:1067–75.

63. Stanchina M, Robinson K, Corrao W, et al. Clinical use of loop gain measures to determine CPAP efficacy in patients with complex sleep apnea: a pilot study. Ann Am Thorac Soc 2015; 12(9):1351–7.

64. Eckert DJ, Owens RL, Kehlmann GB, et al. Eszopiclone increases the respiratory arousal threshold and lowers the apnoea/hypopnoea index in obstructive sleep apnoea patients with a low arousal threshold. Clin Sci (Lond) 2011;120:505–14.

65. Wellman A, Eckert DJ, Jordan AS, et al. A method for measuring and modeling the physiological traits causing obstructive sleep apnea. J Appl Physiol 2011;110:1627–37.

66. Edwards BA, Eckert DJ, McSharry DG, et al. Clinical predictors of the respiratory arousal threshold in patients with obstructive sleep apnea. Am J Respir Crit Care Med 2014;190(11):1293–300.

New Approaches to Positive Airway Pressure Treatment in Obstructive Sleep Apnea

Tomasz J. Kuźniar, MD, PhD

KEYWORDS

- Continuous positive airway pressure • Obstructive sleep apnea • Positive airway pressure
- Compliance

KEY POINTS

- Two basic modes of positive airway pressure – continuous positive airway pressure (CPAP) and autotitrating positive airway pressure (APAP) continue to be the mainstay of therapy in obstructive sleep apnea (OSA).
- Hardware improvements aimed at improving self-sufficiency of patients, and automated adjustments of delivered pressure (Autotrial mode, CPAP check mode) have been introduced.
- Patient comfort features that have been improved include new mask interfaces, improved expiratory pressure relief, heated humidifiers and heated hoses.
- Compliance monitoring has become more effective with wireless transfer of data and online provider and patient-oriented tools.

INTRODUCTION

Continuous positive airway pressure (CPAP) is a mainstay of therapy in patients with obstructive sleep apnea (OSA). Developed in early 1980s,[1] this technology has come over past decades through tremendous changes that resulted in devices that can recognize and differentiate sleep-disordered breathing events, adjust their output to these events, monitor usage, and communicate with the treatment team. This article discusses recent developments in treatment of OSA with PAP.

CONTINUOUS POSITIVE AIRWAY PRESSURE UNITS

Over the years, size and portability of the CPAP device have become key elements of patient's acceptance of therapy. The first CPAPs weighed 6.75 kg; over the years, the device's weight has decreased to 2.5 to 3 lbs, and to less than 1 lb in cases of travel devices. Mirroring the changes in size, the modern CPAP machines have become much quieter than their predecessors. The original CPAP devices were based on vortex blower technology and were so loud that they could be heard several rooms down from the bedroom.[2] Modern devices have advanced motor technology and generate noise as low as 26 dB, less than a whisper, resulting in an improved tolerance of CPAP by patients and their bed partners.

MODES OF CONTINUOUS POSITIVE AIRWAY PRESSURE DELIVERY

Two modes of PAP therapy continue to be used in treatment of patients with OSA. CPAP therapy provides the set pressure, while autotitrating PAP therapy (AutoPAP) devices utilize proprietary

Division of Pulmonary and Critical Care Medicine, NorthShore University HealthSystem, 2650 Ridge Avenue, Evanston, IL 60201, USA
E-mail address: tkuzniar@northshore.org

Sleep Med Clin 11 (2016) 153–159
http://dx.doi.org/10.1016/j.jsmc.2016.03.002
1556-407X/16/$ – see front matter © 2016 Elsevier Inc. All rights reserved.

algorithms to determine presence or absence of obstruction and adjust the pressure generated by the device within the preset range. Although most patients with OSA are treated with set CPAP, AutoPAP devices are used in patients with large sleep stage- or position-related pressure requirements and when in-laboratory titration is unavailable or not effective. Use of these devices is currently not recommended in patients with congestive heart disease, significant chronic lung disease, OSA-independent hypoxemia, central sleep apnea, or in those who do not snore.[3]

AUTOTITRATING POSITIVE AIRWAY PRESSURE

AutoPAP devices use proprietary algorithms to determine the presence/absence of airway obstruction and come up with pressure to resolve it. These algorithms are typically based on the detection of small alterations of flow and pressure patterns, analyzed over a period of time.[4] Although the actual algorithms of PAP devices produced by different manufacturers are not in the public domain, they seem to result in control of airway obstruction at similar pressure and lead to similar treatment outcomes.[5,6]

Phenotypic differences exist between OSA in certain subgroups of patients. For example, female patients seem to be more sensitive to lower degrees of airway flow limitation than male patients. Clinicians now have some degree of control over the type of algorithm on some Auto-PAP devices and can adjust the devices to such subtle phenotypic changes. New Resmed (San Diego, CA) devices allow to choose between a standard "autoset" and an "autoset for her" algorithm that responds faster to small degrees of flow limitation and mildly reduces the time spent with flow limitation in female patients, when compared with the standard algorithm.[7] The DeVilbiss (Somerset, PA) autoadjust algorithm allows one to customize and fine tune the device's response to apneas, hypopneas, and expiratory flow limitation; autoadjust also uniquely allows the detection of expiratory puffs (oral venting).[4]

AUTOTRIAL MODE AND AUTOMATIC PRESSURE ADJUSTMENT (CONTINUOUS POSITIVE AIRWAY PRESSURE CHECK)

AutoPAP algorithm constantly searches for the optimal pressure to maintain airway patency by increasing it in periods of obstruction and decreasing it in periods of good airway control. This, by definition, leads to periods of incomplete control of patency, which may be responsible for incomplete control of sympathetic stimulation by AutoPAP versus CPAP.[8] To address that, switching the device from the "auto" mode to the "set" mode is frequently practiced. Historically, this has been done using the 90th to 95th percentile of pressure generated by the device, based on the download of the compliance card.

This process of transitioning AutoPAP into CPAP can now be done automatically. The autotrial mode, present on Remstar Pro and Remstar Auto devices by Philips Respironics (Murrysville, PA) is equipped with a mode that allows for a smooth, remote transition from autotitrating CPAP to constant pressure CPAP. The autotrial mode, when activated, determines the pressure requirement by the patient, and, after a 30-day period, automatically activates the constant pressure CPAP, set at 90th percentile of pressure determined during the autotrial.[9]

The same Philips Respironics devices are also equipped with a mode that allows dynamic changes in PAP pressure—CPAP check. This mode is most useful on initiation of CPAP pressure or at the end of the 30-day trial of the autotrial mode, described previously. The device, set at a constant CPAP pressure, monitors the effectiveness of obstruction control, and has a capability of automatically rising or lowering the treatment pressure in 1 cmH_2O intervals (and within $\pm$ 3 cmH_2O range from the initial pressure) every 30 hours of use.[10] This allows for adjustments in treatment pressure even prior to the physician follow-up visit.

EXPIRATORY RELIEF

PAP therapy, although primarily aimed at distending the upper airway, has also some effect on the lower airway and chest distension. Physiologically, distension of the chest by CPAP increases the functional residual capacity; exhalation remains a passive event, but it takes place at the higher lung volume than without CPAP. This causes a sensation of incomplete exhalation that is uncomfortable to some CPAP users. Expiratory relief feature is a technology that has been available on CPAP machines since the early 2000s and allows dropping the pressure in the early part of exhalation and helps adjust to this sensation; it may also help with gastric distension.[11] Use of expiratory pressure relief has no effect or may improve PAP compliance, and may be better tolerated than the regular CPAP.[12–14]

How exactly the expiratory relief is produced varies between the manufacturers. Philips Respironics devices are equipped with the digital Auto-Trak system that allows for recognition and compensation of leak, detects the onset of inspiration and expiration, and responds by triggering expiratory pressure relief (flex).[15] Philips' version of expiratory pressure relief comes in 2 variations; C-flex allows for flow-based pressure relief at 3 selectable settings, while C-flex+ offers 3 additional settings for inspiration-to-expiration transition comfort.[15] Similar technology is present on Philips' autotitrating devices (A-flex) and autotitrating bilevel devices.[16,17] Expiratory pressure relief offered on Resmed devices allows dropping of the pressure by a set amount of 1 to 3 cmH$_2$O, which may result in a lower mask leak than in case of C-flex.[18] Similarly, SmartFlex technology on DeVilbiss PAP devices allows one to reduce pressure in 1 cmH$_2$O increments during exhalation; in addition, the inspiratory and expiratory flow rounding technology (6 possible settings) allows for the smooth transition between inspiration and exhalation.[19]

Fisher Paykel (Irvine, CA) devices do not offer an expiratory pressure relief for individual breaths, but rather have SensAwake technology that drops the pressure in periods of irregular breathing associated with wakefulness. This technology lowers the mean pressure generated by the PAP device, without any significant effects on sleep architecture or measures of OSA control.[20]

MASK INTERFACES

Properly fitting and comfortable mask interface are major determinants of CPAP compliance.[21] As the decision to use a particular mask depends on the variety of factors, such as the size and shape of the face, presence of facial hair, size and shape of nostrils, presence of claustrophobia, tendency for nasal/mouth breathing, and even hairstyle, there is not a universally accepted mask interface that will fit every patient. With a multitude of available PAP masks, the old saying that "the best mask for a particular patient is the one that he/she is going to wear" continues to be true.

There has been a considerable advance in mask interfaces since the development of CPAP. Initial PAP masks were made of hard plastic, and in order to assure good fit, had to be custom-made for individual patients. Advances in plastic material technology and introduction of silicone have made them more comfortable and less expensive. Most current masks continue to have a hard plastic shell, with a silicone cuff that is typically removable. They usually come in several sizes, with clear manufacturer recommendations regarding sizing.

There are 3 main classes of PAP masks—nasal, oronasal, and nasal pillows. Comparative data suggest that oronasal masks may be associated with lower compliance with CPAP than 2 other types.[22] However, current trends in interface technology focus on assuring a wide variety of interfaces, allowing the patient to change between models and types of masks. Indeed, adjusting a poor mask fit/changing the mask is the most common intervention performed in a stable patient with OSA.[23]

Over the years, there has been a constant effort to make the interfaces smaller and the headgear less obtrusive. Although prior full-face masks were built with a forehead support plate, several new full mask interfaces (AirFit F10 by Resmed, Amara View by Philips) allow an unobstructed view, which helps in cases of claustrophobia. Also, the design of an exhalation port on current masks reduces the noise produced by escaping air and improves comfort. Finally, recent years have brought simplification of CPAP masks; most current models have a limited number of parts, which makes servicing and cleaning easier than in the case of older, more complex interfaces.

HEATED HUMIDIFICATION

Dry pressurized air may lead to nasal and oropharyngeal dryness, nasal burning or congestion, sneezing and nasal dripping and ultimately cause nocturnal mask slippage and poor compliance.[24] A humidifier unit is now a standard component of any modern CPAP system. Unlike the early in-line, external humidifier systems, modern humidifiers are typically integrated with the CPAP unit. Humidity of the air leaving the humidifier chamber is controlled by the temperature of the heating plate underneath it. Patients are encouraged to adjust the level of humidity to their comfort.

HEATED TUBING

As the warm, humidified air is moved through the hose towards the patient, it is getting colder on contact with the hose. As a result, water may condensate in the tubing and the mask, and cause rainfall from the mask. A tested way of resolving this problem was a thermal insulation that was placed over the hose,[25] minimizing the temperature drop and condensation. Most modern CPAP systems are equipped with a heating wire within the hose itself that helps maintain air temperature and deliver the humidity to the patient (ClimateLine, Resmed; ThermoSmart, Fisher & Paykel; System One Heated Tube, Philips; Heated Tube, DeVilbiss; Hybernite Rainout Control System). Use of the heated tube typically results in an improved nasal patency and sleep quality.[26–28] The temperature of the heating wire is usually controlled separately from the humidifier chamber control. Another layer of the control of humidification is an ambient humidity sensor that measures humidity in the patient's bedroom and adjusts the humidifier output to this level (H5i, Resmed; System One Humidity Control, Philips; ThermoSmart, Fisher & Paykel). This may result in a different usage of water from the humidifier chambers on different nights.[26]

In an effort to minimize the size of PAP equipment, modern humidifier units are smaller than those used in older models. This may limit the amount of water output during the night; at high humidity settings and with the long usage time, the water may be used up by the morning.

COMPLIANCE MONITORING

Compliance with CPAP remains the main barrier to successful treatment of OSA. The advent and popularization of the Internet and increasing ability to obtain, maintain, and transfer large sets of data allowed for rapid development of the technology-rich area of CPAP compliance management. Many of the mechanisms that were introduced to monitor compliance were based on common sense, and their effectiveness has not been formally tested; limited data are available to back up the measurements and interventions that have now become a common practice.

Importantly, the type and amount of data gathered by compliance systems differ between the PAP manufacturers. Also, the nomenclature of detected or calculated parameters differs among manufacturers; 4 most prevalent PAP compliance monitoring systems have different ways of measuring leak, defining a large leak, and detecting and defining apneas and hypopneas.[29] As a result the apnea–hypopnea index (AHI_{Flow}) reported by the compliance systems should not be equated by AHI as measured during sleep studies. A practicing physician needs to have a good understanding of the advantages and deficiencies of particular systems that he or she uses.[29]

Having said that, compliance monitoring is an important component of the everyday practice of sleep medicine. Early CPAP systems were not equipped with a compliance monitor at all; with time, usage hour counters were introduced and then replaced by card-based monitors, that not only registered the usage hours, but also effectiveness of treatment. This technology continues to be used in most PAP devices. Card readers are now typically built into the PAP device, although on some devices, they may have to be externally attached (DeVilbiss PAP devices, SmartLink).[30]

Modern compliance monitoring involves not only a card-based technology, with the card able to store several years' worth of data, but also wireless monitoring. This allows the management team not only to remotely follow the patient's compliance and identify problems, but also to remotely modify the CPAP settings. The new generation of Resmed devices (S10 AirSense and AirCurve) are equipped with a wireless modem that allows for a download of treatment data into a cloud-based compliance tracking system, AirView.[31] It allows for ongoing remote monitoring, and adjustments of treatment parameters. Encore Anywhere is a similar system manufactured by Philips Respironics.

Current insurance regulations require the durable medical equipment (DME) providers to monitor and supply compliance data to the insurers. Wireless technology allowed for retrieval and analysis of large sets of compliance data. U-Sleep,[32] a new monitoring system, extracts the data directly from the AirView and streamlines information on multiple patients. The DME user can set up certain threshold parameters that trigger alerts on noncompliance, lack of effectiveness, mask leakage or other parameters. Signs of usage problems or noncompliance can then be detected and intervened upon early. The software also allows one to group patients with similar types of compliance problems, making interventions on these groups easier. It is also possible to get coaching messages to the patient, based on predefined compliance data parameters, via their favorite communication channel—text message, e-mail, or phone. Finally, U-Sleep also allows patients to access their sleep data, thus promoting patient engagement.

Different technology of compliance monitoring is used in DeVilbiss PAP devices. The device generates an alphanumerical code, which, when entered into the online compliance tool, allows for generation of the compliance report for 1-, 7-, 30-, or 90-day timeframe.[4] This monitoring system requires contact between the user and the provider of the PAP device.

COMPLIANCE MONITORING BY THE PATIENT

Compliance tracking that had started as a physician and device supplier tool has been now made available for patients who are interested in monitoring their treatment. Recognition of the critical role of patient involvement in the successful implementation and continued use of CPAP has led to a rapid growth and development of this area. Higher capacity of data storage and reduced cost of data transmission resulted in the development of software applications that allow the patient to monitor the parameters that were previously only available to the clinicians. Night-to-night feedback with the compliance monitoring system helps maintain motivation and patient's involvement in his or her own treatment.

Sleep Mapper is a mobile- and Web-based free application developed by Philips Respironics that records and reports to the patient a variety of data on daily CPAP usage.[33] Data are then transmitted via an secure digital card (manual download onto a personal computer), Bluetooth, or wireless into a mobile telephone. The application provides daily feedback, allows the patient to set compliance goals, sends the patient reminders regarding CPAP care, and offers educational video materials. Dream Mapper is a newer generation of this software, interfacing with the new generation of Philips Respironics CPAP devices, DreamStation.[34] This new line of devices was expected to be introduced on the US market in late 2015.

New generation of Resmed devices (S10 Airsense and AirCurve) is equipped with a built-in wireless modem that feeds the data into a centralized compliance system. Resmed's version of patient engagement system, MyAir, allows the patient to track the data and tailors coaching to the patient's individual needs.[35]

FUTURE DIRECTIONS OF POSITIVE AIRWAY PRESSURE TREATMENT IN OBSTRUCTIVE SLEEP APNEA

Cost of supervised, in-laboratory polysomnography and low availability of trained sleep medicine specialists have been at the root of the current trend toward less costly, home testing for OSA. Current American Academy of Sleep Medicine guidelines support use of home devices in individuals without significant cardiac or pulmonary comorbidities, and with typical clinical features of OSA. These guidelines have been quickly adopted by a number of private insurers that now only support home diagnostic testing for the majority of patients.

Cost reduction by the payers of health services has also involved the initiation of CPAP therapy. Rather than subjecting the patient to the CPAP titration study, an AutoPAP device is frequently initiated and then adjusted based on the AutoPAP efficacy data. In a recent randomized study, home-based diagnosis of OSA, followed by an AutoPAP therapy, led to a similar effectiveness of therapy, but higher compliance than a laboratory-based diagnosis and PAP titration.[36] Although economically attractive to the payer, this home diagnosis–AutoPAP route was not economically viable to the providers, if the high-quality continuity care was to be maintained.[37] It is now conceivable that much effort will be spent on incorporating new technologies in PAP delivery that allow dynamic changes in the pressure prescription, and intensive monitoring in reducing of the cost and maintaining outcomes of evaluation and treatment of OSA.

Similarly, the high cost of face-to-face contact with the patient will likely increase the role of automated, semiautomated, and remote forms of patient monitoring. Automated telephone-linked communications delivered over the phone by the computer system have been shown to increase patient's adherence to CPAP, compared with no support.[38] Increased patient engagement with therapy of OSA should, as it is the case with other chronic disease, bring an improvement in capability to self-manage one's condition.[39]

Advancements in CPAP technology and monitoring will likely affect provider involvement in routine OSA care. Because most of the need for interventions stemming from a yearly follow-up visit can either be predicted by the presence of specific, subjective complaints from the patient or the analysis of compliance data,[23] it is likely that a routine visit in an OSA patient who is doing well is not needed. This will have to be formally tested.

REFERENCES

1. Sullivan CE, Issa FG, Berthon-Jones M, et al. Reversal of obstructive sleep apnoea by continuous positive airway pressure applied through the nares. Lancet 1981;1(8225):862–5.
2. ResMed. Resmed origins. 2015. Available at: http://www.resmed.com/us/dam/documents/articles/resmed-origins.pdf. Accessed November 1, 2015.
3. Morgenthaler TI, Aurora RN, Brown T, et al. Practice parameters freversal of obstructive sleep apnoea by continuous positive airway pressure applied through the naresor the use of autotitrating continuous positive airway pressure devices for titrating pressures and treating adult patients with obstructive sleep apnea syndrome: an update for 2007. An American academy of sleep medicine report. Sleep 2008; 31(1):141–7.
4. DeVilbiss healthcare. Clinical overview: DeVilbiss IntelliPAP auto adjust. 2014. Available at: http://www.devilbisshealthcare.com/files/LT-2089_RevC_FINAL_050814_Web.pdf. Accessed November 5, 2015.
5. Damiani MF, Quaranta VN, Tedeschi E, et al. Titration effectiveness of two autoadjustable continuous positive airway pressure devices driven by different algorithms in patients with obstructive sleep apnoea. Respirology 2013;18(6):968–73.
6. Senn O, Brack T, Matthews F, et al. Randomized short-term trial of two autoCPAP devices versus fixed continuous positive airway pressure for the treatment of sleep apnea. Am J Respir Crit Care Med 2003;168(12):1506–11.

7. McArdle N, King S, Shepherd K, et al. Study of a novel APAP algorithm for the treatment of obstructive sleep apnea in women. Sleep 2015;38(11):1775–81.

8. Patruno V, Tobaldini E, Bianchi AM, et al. Acute effects of autoadjusting and fixed continuous positive airway pressure treatments on cardiorespiratory coupling in obese patients with obstructive sleep apnea. Eur J Intern Med 2014;25(2):164–8.

9. PhilipsRespironics. Remstar auto with A-flex. Available at: http://www.usa.philips.com/healthcare/product/HCDS560S/system-one-remstar-auto-a-flex. Accessed November 5, 2015.

10. Respironics P. Optimizing CPAP prescription pressures at home. 2012. Available at: http://incenter.medical.philips.com/doclib/enc/9752477/REMstarAutoDataSheetfinal.pdf?func=doc.Fetch&nodeid=9752477. Accessed November 5, 2015.

11. Simmons JH. Treating aerophagia-induced gastric distress (AIGD) associated with CPAP therapy to improve CPAP treatment outcome: understanding the relationship behind oral pressure leakage and AIGD development is key to treatment success. Abstract book. Sleep 2014;37:A108.

12. Aloia MS, Stanchina M, Arnedt JT, et al. Treatment adherence and outcomes in flexible vs standard continuous positive airway pressure therapy. Chest 2005;127:2085–93.

13. Nilius G, Happel A, Domanski U, et al. Pressure-relief continuous positive airway pressure vs constant continuous positive airway pressure: a comparison of efficacy and compliance. Chest 2006;130:1018–24.

14. Chihara Y, Tsuboi T, Hitomi T, et al. Flexible positive airway pressure improves treatment adherence compared with auto-adjusting PAP. Sleep 2013;36(2):229–36.

15. PhilipsRespironics. C-Flex+ pressure relief technology. 2015. Available at: http://www.healthcare.philips.com/main/homehealth/sleep/flexfamily/cflexplus.wpd. Accessed November 4, 2015.

16. Gentina T, Fortin F, Douay B, et al. Auto bi-level with pressure relief during exhalation as a rescue therapy for optimally treated obstructive sleep apnoea patients with poor compliance to continuous positive airways pressure therapy–a pilot study. Sleep Breath 2011;15(1):21–7.

17. Mulgrew AT, Cheema R, Fleetham J, et al. Efficacy and patient satisfaction with autoadjusting CPAP with variable expiratory pressure vs standard CPAP: a two-night randomized crossover trial. Sleep Breath 2007;11(1):31–7.

18. Wolfe LF, Massie CA, Casal E, et al. Comparative efficacy of two expiratory pressure reduction systems in the treatment of obstructive sleep apnea. Sleep Diagn Ther 2009;4(1):1–4.

19. DeVilbiss healthcare. IntelliPAP standard plus with smartflex. 2015. Available at: http://www.devilbisshealthcare.com/products/sleep-therapy/cpap-devices/intellipap-standard-plus. Accessed November 5, 2015.

20. Dungan GC, Marshall NS, Hoyos CM, et al. A randomized crossover trial of the effect of a novel method of pressure control (SensAwake) in automatic continuous positive airway pressure therapy to treat sleep disordered breathing. J Clin Sleep Med 2011;7(3):261–7.

21. Weaver TE. Adherence to positive airway pressure therapy. Curr Opin Pulm Med 2006;12(6):409–13.

22. Borel JC, Tamisier R, Dias-Domingos S, et al. Type of mask may impact on continuous positive airway pressure adherence in apneic patients. PLoS One 2013;8(5):e64382.

23. Nannapaneni S, Morgenthaler TI, Ramar K. Assessing and predicting the likelihood of interventions during routine annual follow-up visits for management of obstructive sleep. J Clin Sleep Med 2014;10(8):919–24.

24. Ulander M, Johansson MS, Ewaldh AE, et al. Side effects to continuous positive airway pressure treatment for obstructive sleep apnoea: changes over time and association to adherence. Sleep Breath 2014;18(4):799–807.

25. Snuggle hose. Available at: http://www.snugglehose.com. Accessed November 1, 2015.

26. Resmed. Humidifier settings. 2015. Available at: http://www.resmed.com/us/en/consumer/support/humidifiers/humidifier-settings-faqs.html. Accessed November 1, 2015.

27. Almasri E, Kline L. The addition of heated wall tubing provides more humidity and comfort than standard humidified CPAP units. Sleep 2007;30(Suppl):A190.

28. Nilius G, Domanski U, Franke K-J, et al. Impact of a controlled heated breathing tube humidifier on sleep quality during CPAP therapy in a cool sleeping environment. Eur Respir J 2008;31(4):830–6.

29. Schwab RJ, Badr SM, Epstein LJ, et al. An official American thoracic society statement: continuous positive airway pressure adherence tracking systems. The optimal monitoring strategies and outcome measures in adults. Am J Respir Crit Care Med 2013;188(5):613–20.

30. DeVilbiss healthcare. Smart link. 2015. Available at: http://www.devilbisshealthcare.com/products/sleep-therapy/therapy-management/smartlink. Accessed November 5, 2015.

31. ResMed. Air view. 2015. Available at: https://airview.resmed.com/login. Accessed November 6, 2015.

32. ResMed. U-sleep. 2015. Available at: http://u-sleep.com. Accessed November 5, 2015.

33. PhilipsRespironics. Sleep mapper. Available at: http://www.usa.philips.com/healthcare-product/HCNOCTN196/sleepmapper. Accessed November 5, 2015.

34. PhilipsRespironics. Dream mapper. 2015. Available at: https://www.sleepapnea.com/products/dream mapper/. Accessed October 21, 2015.

35. ResMed. My air. 2015. Available at: http://www.resmed.com/us/en/healthcare-professional/air-solutions/patient-engagement/myair.html. Accessed November 6, 2015.

36. Rosen CL, Auckley D, Benca R, et al. A multisite randomized trial of portable sleep studies and positive airway pressure autotitration versus laboratory-based polysomnography for the diagnosis and treatment of obstructive sleep apnea: the HomePAP study. Sleep 2012;35(6):757–67.

37. Kim RD, Kapur VK, Redline-Bruch J, et al. An economic evaluation of home versus laboratory-based diagnosis of obstructive sleep apnea. Sleep 2015; 38(07):1027–37.

38. Sparrow D, Aloia M, Demolles DA, et al. A telemedicine intervention to improve adherence to continuous positive airway pressure: a randomised controlled trial. Thorax 2010;65(12):1061–6.

39. Coulter A, Entwistle VA, Eccles A, et al. Personalised care planning for adults with chronic or long-term health conditions. Cochrane Database Syst Rev 2015;(3):CD010523.

Monitoring Progress and Adherence with Positive Airway Pressure Therapy for Obstructive Sleep Apnea
The Roles of Telemedicine and Mobile Health Applications

Dennis Hwang, MD

KEYWORDS

- CPAP adherence • CPAP follow-up • Telemedicine • Self-management • Patient engagement
- Mobile health applications • Wearable sensors • Electronic health records

KEY POINTS

- Telemedicine and its integration into the overall health technology ecosystem is a critical component of the evolving solution for obstructive sleep apnea management and continuous positive airway pressure (CPAP) adherence.
- Current strategies that can be practically implemented include the use of Web-education, adoption of automated and self-management CPAP follow-up platforms, and providing patients information regarding online support groups.
- The future holds unlimited possibilities, from the expansion of mobile health applications and wearable sensors to electronic health record integration that can streamline end-to-end comprehensive care and provide advanced analytics to enhance disease management and facilitate population health management.

INTRODUCTION

The world is changing. Technology is now integral to most aspects of the day-to-day lives for people in the United States, and this is true also of health care. In 2015, the *Wall Street Journal* published an article titled, "The Future of Medicine is in Your Smartphone."[1] Although this title is largely projecting into tomorrow, it is evident that the responsibilities of health care providers and the way that patients approach their health are already substantially evolving. From the widespread adoption of electronic health records (EHRs), to the ubiquitous nature of smartphone and health applications, to the increasing proliferation of wearable devices, it is clear that medicine must figure how to embrace technology and use it to the benefit of medical providers, the global health system, and ultimately for patients.

Disclosure Statement: The author has received recent research support from the American Sleep Medicine Foundation (ASMF; Physician Scientist Training Award and Strategic Research grant 104SR13) and Itamar Medical Ltd. The author has previously received research support from the National Institutes of Health (grant 1 T32 HL072752) and Ventus Medical, Inc. ASMF supported the research presented on **Fig. 1**. The other sponsors do not represent a conflict of interest.
Sleep Medicine, Southern California Permanente Medical Group, Kaiser Permanente Fontana Sleep Disorders Center, 9961 Sierra Avenue, Fontana, CA 92335, USA
E-mail address: Dennis.x.hwang@kp.org

Sleep Med Clin 11 (2016) 161–171
http://dx.doi.org/10.1016/j.jsmc.2016.01.008
1556-407X/16/$ – see front matter

It is well documented that a major challenge for sleep specialists is optimizing adherence of patients with obstructive sleep apnea (OSA) to continuous positive airway pressure (CPAP) therapy. Literature generally reports that only half of patients remain adherent to CPAP 3 months after initiating therapy.[2] Efforts to improve adherence through advances in CPAP technology have not proven fruitful, whereas psychosocial interventions are often labor intensive and modest in effect. Given the impact of OSA on a person's overall well-being and on the public health system, it is imperative to successfully answer the following question: How can technology be a solution to the problem of CPAP adherence? The goal of this article is to explore sleep medicine's approach toward addressing this issue. The author provides a general overview of health-related technologies while clarifying the scope of telemedicine, discusses current and emerging sleep medicine telemedicine platforms, and understands the evolution of the health information technology (health IT) ecosystem and its anticipated impact on sleep medicine.

OVERVIEW OF TELEMEDICINE
Definitions

Telemedicine is key to improving our ability to care for patients with OSA. However, there is confusion regarding the meaning of telemedicine, and clarifying its definition and purview is necessary to create a framework for the overall discussion within this article. There are 2 basic types of telemedicine, synchronous and asynchronous. *Synchronous* refers to mechanisms in which medical care is delivered in real-time, and this includes video visits, which are often incorrectly used synonymously with telemedicine. Video visits may be useful for sleep medicine for several reasons:

1. Limits travel time for frequently sleepy patients
2. Expands the geographic area, particularly remote areas, in which a sleep specialist can provide care
3. Enhances CPAP education and troubleshooting over a simple telephone call because of the ability to visually assess and demonstrate mask fit and equipment use

In the author's sleep center, the use of video visits has expanded from sleep physicians to respiratory therapists (to provide CPAP troubleshooting); both patient and provider experience has been overwhelmingly positive. The American Academy of Sleep Medicine has recognized the value of expanding video visits within this field. It convened a task force that published a position paper aimed at assisting sleep specialists in incorporating video visit capabilities into their practice: "American Academy of Sleep Medicine (AASM) Position Paper for the Use of Telemedicine for the Diagnosis and Treatment of Sleep Disorders".[3]

The limitation of synchronous telemedicine, however, is that it still requires face-to-face provider time. The American Telemedicine Association states that the 3 primary goals of telemedicine are to (1) improve access to care, (2) improve quality of care, and (3) improve efficiency or cost-effectiveness of care.[4] Although video visits can improve access and quality of care, its impact on care efficiency is modest at best. Rather, in order to do so, it requires the adoption of elements that largely fall under the purview of *asynchronous* telemedicine.

Asynchronous Telemedicine

Overview
Asynchronous telemedicine, also called store-and-forward, indicates that the encounter between patients and provider does not occur in real-time. Examples of this include the following:

- Electronic messaging: the use of e-mail and text messaging to communicate with patients or deliver medical information
- Remote monitoring: (1) accessing stored patient data from a medical test and reviewing at a later time from a remote location (eg, sleep physicians accessing polysomnography [PSG] data for interpretation) and (2) accessing patient-collected data from end-user devices, including wireless access of data from patients' home medical devices (eg, Glucometers, sphygmomanometer, CPAP devices) or data from personal mobile devices (eg, smartphones, tablets) that often have installed health applications or are linked to a wearable sensor
- Automated care mechanisms and self-management platforms: (1) platforms that automate patient feedback based on therapy adherence and (2) smartphone applications (often with wearable sensors) that can provide a continuous system of accountability

These elements are *key principles* that underpin the ability of asynchronous mechanisms to improve the efficiency of care delivery and are evident in the eventual discussion on sleep telemedicine platforms relevant to OSA management. For now, each of these principles is further explored.

Electronic messaging
Virtually all patients have access to e-mail and text messaging. In a research study performed in the

author's center, 556 patients were given the choice to receive feedback regarding their CPAP use by phone call, e-mail, or text messaging. Only 4% chose phone call, thus, reflecting a shift in patient attitudes regarding their preferred method of communicating with medical providers (D. Hwang, unpublished data, 2015). The use of messaging has been demonstrated to be effective. A research study (The Tobacco, Exercise and Diet Messages trial) randomized patients with cardiovascular risk factors into an intervention group that received 4 automated text messages (providing advice and motivational reminders to adhere to lifestyle changes) each week for 6 months. When compared with controls, lipid profiles (low-density lipoprotein), blood pressure, body mass index, and smoking rates were all significantly lower at 6 months, whereas the amount of weekly physical activity was higher.[5] Another study found that 91% of patients who were regularly and automatically sent text messages were adherent to hypertensive medication compared with 75% of controls.[6] These studies demonstrate how electronic messaging with automated delivery can be effective at improving patient engagement and therapy adherence. Later in this article, the author discusses how this can also be used to improve CPAP utilization.

Remote monitoring

The widespread availability of cellular networks and home Wi-Fi networks is enhancing accessibility of medical information, particularly data that are stored by patients' medical and personal devices. Simply being able to access data that are actionable can be potentially effective. In one study, a group of patients received a Bluetooth-enabled blood pressure cuff that enabled medical providers to review readings weekly. If the blood pressure was greater than the goal, patients would be called; this resulted in an improvement in blood pressure at 6 months. (Systolic blood pressure improved by an average of 13 mm Hg compared with 8.5 mm Hg in the control group.)[7] The impact of remote monitoring is particularly relevant given the wireless capabilities of new-generation CPAP devices.

Automated and self-management mechanisms

Automated electronic messaging is one example of automated care mechanisms. Another example is technology that empowers patients to care for themselves, such as through the use of mobile health applications and wearable sensors. The popularity of these technologies is exploding. There were nearly 20,000 medical applications available in the Apple application store in 2013, and 21% of people in the United States owned a

wearable device as of 2014.[8] Although actual randomized controlled studies demonstrating the effectiveness of these interventions are not yet available, anecdotal experience is filled with examples of how these technologies have changed lives. MyFitnessPal (MyFitnessPal Inc, San Francisco, CA), which is a diet and exercise diary program, has helped several people lose significant weight. FitBit (FitBit Inc, San Francisco, CA), which is a wrist-worn activity tracker, has helped many people improve their level of physical activity. These self-management platforms include the ability to provide near-constant accountability (whereas provider-based follow-up is intermittent and relatively infrequent), and they are vehicles to delivering education and information enabling patients to self-troubleshoot issues with their therapy. Similar principles can be applied that may be potentially useful in engaging patients with CPAP.

SLEEP MEDICINE AND TELEMEDICINE
Overview

The author has provided an overview of telemedicine and its various components. In this section, the author discusses the development of sleep-specific telemedicine platforms while recognizing the underlying key principles discussed in the previous section. Sleep medicine is a field that relies heavily on technology. As mentioned earlier, sleep specialists have been able to digitally review PSG data in real-time (and take manual control of therapy titrations) or after study completion. Many home sleep apnea testing (HSAT) devices have remote capabilities in which study data can be uploaded into a cloud server and accessible from any location with Internet access. One platform (NovaSom) will actually directly transmit the data via cellular service directly from the device into their server without the need for a medical provider to manually upload.

As the health care environment is evolving to reward clinical outcomes rather than for services provided, implementing cost-effective care management solutions is critical. One example whereby sleep telemedicine has been shown to be effective is the use of Internet or mobile-based cognitive behavioral therapy programs for insomnia, which can provide tools for self-management and provide daily and continuous accountability.[9] The question explored here is whether similar platforms exist for managing OSA and improving CPAP adherence. Psychosocial interventions have had some impact, specifically through enhancing patient education and providing intensive follow-up; but both these approaches tend to be very labor intensive. In this section, whether technology can be a cost-effective solution to delivering these strategies is explored further.

Telemedicine and Obstructive Sleep Apnea Education

Patient education is foundational to getting patients engaged with therapy; but the optimal format, information, and delivery mechanism is unclear. An extensive educational program was evaluated that involved 36 hours of attendance to an outpatient program that included (1) comprehensive daytime OSA and CPAP education, (2) group session with inclusion of spouses, (3) focused workshops, and (4) individualized discussion.[10] Despite this intensive education, the impact on CPAP use at 3 months was small, resulting in a nonstatistically significant improvement in CPAP use by an average of 0.7 hours per night in a cohort of 35 patients. Even if we assume a real difference is evident, it is clear that the program was labor intensive with minimal impact. The question is whether technology-based delivery of education can be a more cost-effective solution.

One study evaluated the use of a 15-minute CPAP educational video at the time of therapy initiation.[11] In a randomized trial, those who viewed the video did demonstrate improved patient engagement when measuring the rate in which the patients kept their 1-month follow-up appointment (73% vs 49%; $P = .02$). They were reported to be more likely to use CPAP, although actual CPAP use was not published and was limited by incomplete available usage data (one reason was the incomplete rate of follow-up).

Despite uncertain benefits on CPAP adherence, telemedicine-delivered education is likely an essential component in developing OSA clinical care pathways. In choosing from the various available OSA educational platforms, programs should ideally include the following components: (1) remote electronic delivery, (2) personalized invitations, (3) interactive, (4) viewable on demand and as many times as desired, and (5) concise and easy to understand. Emmi Solutions is one company that specializes in Internet-based medical education that includes those characteristics; they have developed a diverse set of OSA educational programs: OSA education, CPAP education, and sleep study preparation education. An unscientific survey of the patients in the author's center provided feedback on Emmi:

- Ninety-three percent stated it answered a question they otherwise would have called their physician to ask.
- Ninety-three percent stated they would take new action in managing their health.
- Ninety percent felt more positively toward our health care organization.

A randomized trial evaluating the impact of Emmi is discussed later in this article. Although it is unlikely that automated educational processes can completely replace face-to-face education, its value as an adjunct educational platform is probably quite significant.

Telemedicine and Continuous Positive Airway Pressure Follow-up

Overview

The use of telemedicine to enhance CPAP follow-up is the area that has been the most explored. Intensive support after CPAP initiation clearly improves use. In patients who underwent an intensive support program (CPAP education in patients' homes that included the patients' partners; nurse home visits at 4 time points over 6 months), 6-month CPAP use was better compared with controls (5.4 vs 3.9 hours per night; $P = .0003$).[12] This protocol is again limited by its labor intensiveness, and the question is whether using telemedicine as the support system can be less costly and more effective.

Initial forays into the use of telecommunications for facilitating follow-up included the use of interactive voice response (IVR), which is a telephone mechanism to survey patients. IVR can automate calls to patients and ask a series of questions formatted in a way so that patients can answer by pushing the telephone keypad, for example: Are you using CPAP? Press 1 for yes, press 2 for no. How many days this week did you use your CPAP? In one study of 30 patients, IVR was used to ask patients questions regarding their CPAP use. If the use was suboptimal based on predetermined thresholds, the system would proceed to ask questions aimed at identifying the cause, then provide brief education and reinforce regular CPAP use. Those randomized to IVR had a trend toward improved use at 2 months compared with controls (4.4 vs 2.9 hours per night; $P = .08$).[13] A subsequent trial of 250 patients demonstrated that those supported with IVR had higher usage at 6 months and 12 months by 1 and 2 hours per night, respectively, compared with controls. In this study, the intervention-group patients were expected to make weekly calls into the IVR call-in system during the first month and then monthly until the year was complete. If patients missed their scheduled call-in, the IVR system would automatically call the patients.

Limitations on using IVR as described in these studies include the following: (1) Reviewing IVR results is still a labor-intensive process. The larger

IVR study did not report the number of provider hours used to provide follow-up based on their protocol, but the author's own experience using IVR for CPAP follow-up was excessively labor intensive because of having to manually review copious amounts of IVR data for a large cohort of patients. (2) Reliance on patients to self-report their CPAP use is a limitation, and literature has indicated that patients tend to overestimate actual use.[2] The ability to remotely access *objective* CPAP data was enabled by a technology that emerged in the mid-2000s, which proved to be a game changer for sleep medicine: cellular wireless capability.

Wireless transfer of continuous positive airway pressure data

Various CPAP modems have been developed that include enabling the use of wired Ethernet cable, home Wi-Fi networks, and Bluetooth connections to transfer data to a cloud database. The largest CPAP vendors, however, are moving toward using cellular connection as the standard. The key advantage of this technology is that the individual's CPAP data are now automatically collected, remotely accessible, and actionable by both providers and patients.

In 2007, Stepnowsky and colleagues[14] performed a study in which 45 patients were randomized into a remote monitoring pathway or usual care. The remote monitoring protocol included manual access by the sleep specialists to review hours of use, mask leak, and apnea hypopnea index (AHI). Usual care involved a 1-week telephone encounter and a 1-month follow-up office visit. A trend was evident that remote monitoring improved CPAP use at 2 months compared with usual care (4.1 vs 2.8 hours per night; $P = .07$). A similar study of 75 patients who also used remote monitoring demonstrated near doubling of CPAP use at 3 months (191 vs 105 minutes per night; $P = .006$).[15] In this study, a research coordinator monitored CPAP data on a daily basis, and then a clinical case manager contacted the patients if CPAP data indicated suboptimal use or other problems. Although availability of objective and diverse CPAP data enables more useful and actionable information, it suffers from the same limitation as IVR in that it leads to data overload when trying to manage a large patient population. The latter study quantified provider time and found that an additional 67 minutes on average per patient was spent managing the patients that were remotely monitored. Considering the near doubling of CPAP use, this still may be cost-effective even if labor intensive. It should be noted that the study follow-up period was limited to 3 months, and the effect on long-term compliance remains unknown. In order to extend remote monitoring indefinitely and to do so efficiently, implementing automated mechanisms and self-management programs are necessary.

Automated mechanisms and self-management continuous positive airway pressure follow-up platforms

The ability to automatically transmit CPAP data is not only useful when accessible by the sleep specialist but also when accessible by patients. Just the mere availability of this data for patients to access on their own has been shown to improve CPAP adherence. Kuna and colleagues[16] performed a study of 138 patients randomized to *usual care* and *usual care with patient access to CPAP data via an online portal*. Those with access had significantly better CPAP use per night (about 6 hours) compared with usual care (4.7 hours) at the 3-month follow-up. Patient log-ins were noted to drastically decline after the first week, although the improved CPAP use was maintained throughout the 3-month period. This study demonstrated that mere access to their own data can improve patient adherence; but the authors did note that addition of a self-management program (ie, self-troubleshooting information, reward system) might better sustain patient engagement even beyond the first week.

The first dedicated CPAP self-management platform that used wirelessly transmitted CPAP data may have been a platform called MyCPAP, which was tested at the University of California, San Diego (UCSD).[17] MyCPAP was a Web site that included the following components:

1. Learning center: provided basic education regarding OSA and CPAP
2. CPAP data: provided patient access to their usage and efficacy information in the form of charts
3. Surveys: provided questionnaires to assess subjective symptoms, which was then tracked over time in graphs
4. Troubleshooting guide: provided an interactive guide that would direct patients to learn about possible solutions to their identified CPAP problem
5. User's manual: provided education regarding how to use and care for CPAP and accessories

In a randomized trial of 241 patients, those who participated in MyCPAP had significantly improved CPAP use at 2 months compared with controls (4.1 vs 3.4 hours per night; $P = .02$). Although the frequency of log-ins were not recorded, patients in the intervention group indicated a greater frequency of using the Internet to search medical information at study completion than at baseline, suggesting that this surrogate metric may reflect that engagement with MyCPAP improved over time (unlike the fall-off seen in the study by Kuna and colleagues[16] after the first week.)

Current Sleep Telemedicine Solutions

This article, up to this point, focuses on developing the framework of telemedicine while describing the background evolution of sleep telemedicine technologies. But where are we today? What platforms are currently available for adoption? Self-management and automated solutions have continued to evolve and are now largely developed and maintained by CPAP vendors. CPAP companies have expanded from being primarily a device company to one that aims to be a comprehensive OSA solution that includes diagnostic testing devices and expansion of follow-up strategies.

Philips Respironics developed a self-management platform in the form of a mobile device application called DreamMapper (previously called SleepMapper). This platform mimics the UCSD MyCPAP program in that it presents patients their CPAP data in easy-to-track graphs and provides CPAP troubleshooting material while also creating a reward system to encourage use. SleepMapper functions by using data transferred from patients' CPAP to an online database called EncoreAnywhere. In a retrospective review of their entire EncoreAnywhere database of about 15,000 patients, they were able to identify patients that *used* and *did not use* SleepMapper for comparison.[18] Seventy-eight percent of those who used SleepMapper were compliant at 90 days (Medicare definition) compared with 56% of those who did not, and they used CPAP for an average of 1.4 hours longer per night. The limitation with this study is the retrospective noncontrolled nature of these data with significant potential confounding factors. Patients who volunteered to use SleepMapper are likely naturally more engaged with CPAP use even independent of SleepMapper.

ResMed Corp also has their own follow-up solution. Their most updated CPAP devices are now all equipped with an active cellular modem, and virtually all these patients have access to their CPAP data through a portal called MyAir, which also includes a self-management system. This portal can be accessed via an Internet browser or a mobile device application (available on both the Apple store and Google Play). Another ResMed follow-up solution is called U-Sleep. One of its main functions is to provide active feedback by processing CPAP data (that is automatically and remotely collected), followed by sending

automated messages encouraging use back to the patients when their CPAP usage is suboptimal or other problems are identified. A recent study randomized 120 new CPAP users into usual care (4 telephone follow-up over 3 months) or U-Sleep without the scheduled telephone encounters.[19] The U-Sleep patients did have better CPAP usage at 3 months (83% vs 73% Medicare compliance), but the difference was not statistically significant. Rather, the primary finding is that fewer coaching minutes were required during the 3-month follow-up period for the U-Sleep versus usual-care patients (24 vs 58 minutes; $P<.0001$). The suggestion is that U-Sleep may be a cost-effective solution by potentially replacing traditional scheduled follow-up protocols without drop-off in CPAP adherence.

The author has discussed telemedicine mechanisms that address different psychosocial targets: (1) delivery of education and (2) implementing automated follow-up system. Telemedicine mechanisms have been discussed that target different psychosocial targets. Would adding these mechanisms together sequentially within an episode of care have a synergistic effect? In other words, would Web-OSA education added to an automated CPAP follow-up program impact CPAP adherence to a greater degree than either of those platforms used in isolation? The author's center performed a 4-arm randomized controlled trial of 1873 patients evaluating the impact of Emmi Web-education and U-Sleep.[20] Web-education entailed sending patients an Emmi education program on OSA 1 week before their sleep study appointment. If patients had OSA, another Emmi program focused on CPAP education was sent during the patients' first-week CPAP trial. In this study, patients were randomized into (1) usual care (3-month follow-up), (2) usual care plus Emmi, (3) usual care plus U-Sleep, and (4) usual care plus Emmi and U-Sleep. The results demonstrated a stepwise increase in CPAP compliance that was greatest in those who received both Emmi and U-Sleep (**Fig. 1**). However, the increase in CPAP use was statistically significant only for U-Sleep versus no U-Sleep (70% vs 58%; $P<.01$), which represents a 21% improvement. Although Emmi did not significantly improve CPAP adherence (66% vs 59%; $P = .09$), Emmi did improve patient adherence in keeping their sleep study appointment (68% vs 63%; $P = .04$). This study demonstrated different but complementary benefits when using telemedicine to target 2 different components of care delivery. Additional telemedicine mechanisms that target expanded care components are emerging, and their potential impact on OSA management is explored in this next section.

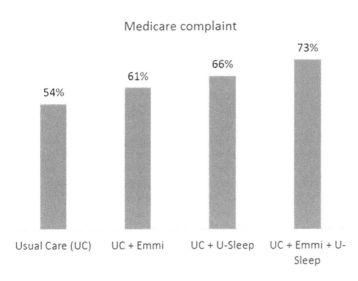

Medicare complaint

54% 61% 66% 73%

Usual Care (UC)   UC + Emmi   UC + U-Sleep   UC + Emmi + U-Sleep

Fig. 1. CPAP compliance was greatest in those who received Emmi and U-Sleep. Difference compared with UC + U-Sleep was not statistically significant.

HEALTH INFORMATION TECHNOLOGY: THE DEVELOPING ECOSYSTEM
Overview

As discussed earlier in the article, the purview of telemedicine is wide, but current strategies are currently limited. The author's discussion of current technologies has focused primarily on enhancing automated follow-up mechanisms and delivery of educational material. In order to understand additional capabilities of using technology to enhance the sleep specialist's ability to manage OSA requires understanding the greater context of the health technology ecosystem and how it is evolving.

The health information technology (IT) ecosystem is rapidly expanding, both in regard to peripheral consumer-based devices as well as central provider-based technologies. Furthermore, it is not only expanding but it is also rapidly coalescing into a developing streamlined infrastructure. In other words, the various technology components are not developing in isolation. Rather they are interconnecting and integrating. In this next section, the author discusses a few emerging trends in the world of health IT that may enhance the way sleep specialists manage patients with OSA.

Sleep Mobile Device Applications and Wearable Sensors

Background
Telemedicine solutions discussed up to this point have primarily been provider-based. There is, however, an on-going shift in health care from being provider centric to one that reflects increased ownership by patients; this is reflected in the increased use of consumer-driven mobile health applications and wearable sensors. As previously mentioned, one-fifth of Americans in 2014 owned a wearable device, such as a FitBit; the prevalence continues to increase.[21] The popularity has increased to the point that *Consumer Reports* has a section dedicated to rating available fitness trackers.[22]

One of the key uses of these devices has been to measure not only physical activity but to also measure sleep. Although the accuracy of sleep data requires further validation and the proper uses of these devices requires additional exploration, the prevalence of these device warrants the sleep specialist to understand the current evidence in order to have educated discussions with patients. It is now commonplace for sleep specialists to encounter patients in clinic armed with sleep data collected from one of these devices.

Types of devices
Multiple kinds of devices are available, such as smart watches, activity tracking belts, shoes that measure running distance and speed, skin patches that measure ultraviolet ray exposure, and earbuds that can respond to commands.[23] The most popular wearable devices are worn on the wrist and track activity through accelerometers that sense motion (as well as measure lack of motion). These devices usually connect wirelessly to a software application on patients' mobile devices (ie, smartphone) that processes the data and reports it back to patients. Some applications are not linked to a wearable device but rather use the native accelerometer on patients' smartphones. One popular application called Sleep Cycle involves placing the smartphone near the end of the bed to track movements during sleep and produces graphs portraying patterns of sleep (light and deep sleep) and wake periods. There is also a function that will adjust the alarm

time to activate only when the person is not in deep sleep in order to limit postwake grogginess. It should be noted that a similar application called Sleep Time was compared with PSG, and the sleep parameters (sleep efficiency, light sleep, deep sleep) showed no correlation.[24]

On the other end of the spectrum, some devices claim more complex sleep-related functions. One company produces headphones studded with sensors and asserts the ability to sense deep sleep and induce lucid dreaming with the goal of improving sleep quality.[25] Others are emerging that attempt to evaluate the risk of OSA by measuring parameters associated with snoring or integrate more complex signals, such as electro-encephalogram, oxygen saturation, and cardiac signals. But the use of these more advanced wearables is mostly nonvalidated and not as common as those focused on tracking activity, such as Fit-Bit and similar devices.

Activity trackers

Activity trackers are essentially simple acceler-ometers that send motion data to a software application, which then processes the data to determine wake and sleep periods, similar to that of traditional sleep actigraphy devices. Several wrist-worn devices are commercially available; FitBit and JawBone are 2 of the more common ones. A recent review of 22 studies evaluating wearable activity trackers concluded that they were better at measuring physical activity (specifically number of steps) than measuring sleep.[26] Only 4 studies were available (FitBit and Jawbone) that compared these trackers with PSG, and they indicated that these devices generally overestimate sleep (total sleep time and sleep efficiency) while underestimating wake. FitBit does have an ultrasensitive mode that reverses this and underestimates sleep while overestimating wake.[27]

Practical implications

It is important for the sleep specialist to understand the evidence, albeit limited, regarding wearables. One 16-year-old patient came into the author's center for a PSG because her mother thought her FitBit was reporting a sleep problem. Her PSG was normal, and her history indicated normal sleep pattern and daytime vigilance. The mother insisted that a sleep problem was present, and it was only the ability to conduct an educated discussion based on published data that the family was reassured. On the other hand, these devices can function as a crude screening mechanism. Anec-dotal experience also describes patients whose wearable device indicates a sleep problem and properly seek out a sleep specialist for a diagnosis.

It is important for sleep medicine to explore how these devices can be best incorporated into sleep medicine work flow given their increasing popularity, continuing advancements in their functions, and their evident ability to engage patients. Perhaps these devices can be validated as a formal OSA screening mechanism or track improvements in sleep after initiating CPAP therapy. Maybe devices with advanced functions (ie, oximetry) can be used to identify when patients with chronic hypercapnic respiratory failure on noninvasive ventilation are beginning to decompensate, providing an opportunity to intervene before requiring hospitalization. The world of wearables is here to stay, and our job is to figure out how to unlock the unlimited possibilities.

Peer-Based Follow-up

Peer-based follow-up is another promising follow-up strategy that has been explored in conditions, such as human immunodeficiency virus, heart failure, and diabetes.[28] Although it does not represent a new unique technology, it does typically use telecommunications and the Internet to facilitate this form of self-directed care. Parthsarathy and colleagues[29] published a pilot study in 2013 in which 39 patients were randomized into a buddy system or to usual care. The buddy system involved matching new CPAP users to an experienced CPAP user who would effectively act as a mentor over 3 months. After 2 face-to-face sessions, the mentor would call the new user weekly for 1 month and then every 2 weeks. Ninety-one percent of patients found the experience to be satisfactory, and measures of CPAP adherence were overall better in patients who were mentored (64% of patients in the buddy system were considered adherent compared with 40% in the usual-care group.) Although feasibility of a buddy system in a standard sleep center requires further investigation, other peer-based programs already do exist in the form of Internet group forums, which can provide peer-based engagement, additional education, and motivational testimonials. Examples of these online communities are hosted by the American Sleep Apnea Association, MyApnea.org (which also functions as a patient-driven research platform), and a ResMed portal called WakeUpToSleep.com.

Electronic Health Records and Technology Integration

General concepts

EHRs have become an integral component of the health care system in the United States. It has the potential to transform medicine through its ability to enhance provider documentation, share data between providers and patients, extend medical care by enabling remote and automated functions, and facilitate data analytics. Current use of EHRs, however, is primarily limited to provider documentation and as a repository for results, such as laboratory, radiography, and other medical tests, including sleep studies. As previously discussed, the health IT ecosystem is coalescing into an infrastructure of interconnecting peripheral patient end-user devices (personal devices and prescribed therapies, such as CPAP) and EHRs, which represents the center of the health IT ecosystem. Health IT integration is fundamentally the connecting of telemedicine mechanisms into EHR. This section further explores the potential of EHR integration and how it can transform the ability to care for patients with OSA.

Device integration

Because of multiple sleep diagnostic and therapy devices used in sleep medicine, sleep specialists are challenged by having to operate within several interfaces and by encumbered transfer of sleep study results into patients' charts. Integration of sleep devices (PSG, HSAT, CPAP) with EHRs addresses these challenges in the following ways:

1. It enables automatic and efficient transfer of sleep data.
2. It improves user experience. The data from multiple devices can be viewed by the sleep provider in one interface rather than a different interface for each sleep device used.
3. The data retain their discrete value and can be processed. Current transfer of sleep study data into EHR is primarily a copy-paste mechanism in which the data are transferred in a text format. This mechanism limits the ability to process that information needed to facilitate automated care mechanisms, data analytics, and enhanced provider documentation. For example, the AHI metric that retains its numerical value can be used for population health management (described later), whereas CPAP data can also be efficiently imported into a provider clinic note through a shortcut mechanism to make documentation more efficient.

Tablets used to survey patients (ie, sleep scales and intake questionnaires) can also be integrated with EHRs, which enables transfer of survey results with discrete values, thus, sharing these similar advantages.

Data analytics: population health management

Availability of discrete data is powerful because it can be processed to facilitate critical elements of care delivery, including (1) screening for risk of sleep and nonsleep disorders, (2) predictive analytics to assist in clinical decision making for individual patients, and (3) querying clinical outcomes. Querying outcomes can be useful for reporting to payers, tracking service quality metrics, and for research; these elements are further discussed in this issue (see Budhiraja R, Thomas R, Kim M, et al: The Role of Big Data in the Management of Sleep-Disordered Breathing). Querying outcomes can also directly assist care delivery because it is the engine that drives population health management. Population management is the application of select actionable items identified by analyzing a wide range of clinical data to an aggregate group of patients defined by similar characteristics.[30] The goal is to enhance the efficiency and effectiveness of improving health outcomes for that group by monitoring and managing individuals within that group with select characteristics. For example, EHRs can automatically compile a set of patients with severe OSA and suboptimal CPAP use 1 month after initiating therapy. These patients can be prioritized for troubleshooting with the goal of improving outcomes for that select cohort.

Work flow integration: clinical care pathways

EHR integration cannot only streamline core components of care (diagnostic testing, therapy initiation, and immediate follow-up care) but it can also tie in the outer ends of the end-to-end care spectrum (**Fig. 2**). As discussed, the core components of care can be enhanced by device integration that enables automatic transfer of diagnostic and therapy data that is actionable. At the early end of the spectrum, EHRs can screen individual patients or a select population of patients (ie, preoperative patients); it can automatically send Web-education programs and intake questionnaires linked to a scheduled sleep clinic appointment. At the other end of the spectrum, EHRs can be linked to automated follow-up platforms to provide continuous and indefinite remote monitoring and facilitate ongoing population management as previously described. Eventually, integration of wearable sensors may be able to add further actionable data that can potentially facilitate disease management across specialties. For example, patients with congestive heart failure can be monitored by wearables that can detect decreases in oxygen saturation, increases in irregular heart rhythms, and increases in body weight in addition to a CPAP device demonstrating an increase in

Care Component

EHR Function

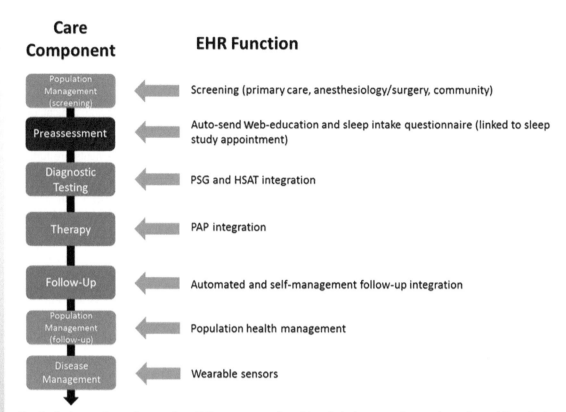

Screening (primary care, anesthesiology/surgery, community)

Auto-send Web-education and sleep intake questionnaire (linked to sleep study appointment)

PSG and HSAT integration

PAP integration

Automated and self-management follow-up integration

Population health management

Wearable sensors

Fig. 2. End-to-end care integration: EHRs can streamline OSA clinical care pathways through enabling device integration (sleep devices, follow-up platforms, wearable sensors), facilitating patient-provider interchange (questionnaires, Web education), and advanced data analytics (screening, population management).

periodic breathing. The medical provider can be alerted to impending decompensation and provide an opportunity to intervene before hospitalization. EHRs, in conjunction with a progressively integrated network of telemedicine technologies, can potentially revolutionize the way sleep specialists manage OSA with increasing relevance across specialties and to patients.

SUMMARY

Telemedicine and its integration into the overall health technology ecosystem is a critical component of the evolving solution for OSA management and CPAP adherence. Current strategies that can be practically implemented include the use of Web-education, adoption of automated and self-management CPAP follow-up platforms, and providing patients information regarding online support groups. The future, however, holds unlimited possibilities, from the expansion of mobile health applications and wearable sensors to EHR integration that can streamline end-to-end comprehensive care and provide advanced analytics to facilitate population health management

and predictive analytics. The world is changing indeed; tomorrow is just around the corner.

REFERENCES

1. Topol EJ. The future of medicine is in your smartphone. Wall Street Journal 2015. Available at: http://www.wsj.com/articles/the-future-of-medicine-is-in-your-smartphone-1420828632. Accessed October 15, 2015.
2. Kribbs NB, Pack AI, Kline LR, et al. Objective measurement of patterns of nasal CPAP use by patients with obstructive sleep apnea. Am Rev Respir Dis 1993;147(4):887–95.
3. Singh J, Badr SM, Hwang D, et al. American Academy of Sleep Medicine (AASM) position paper for the use of telemedicine for the diagnosis and treatment of sleep disorders. J Clin Sleep Med 2015; 11(10):1187–98.
4. What is Telemedicine? Available at: http://www.americantelemed.org/about-telemedicine/what-is-telemedicine#.VpwOjxUrLuo. Accessed October 15, 2015.
5. Chow CK, Redfern J, Hillis GS, et al. Effect of lifestyle-focused text messaging on risk factor

modification in patients with coronary heart disease. JAMA 2015;314(12):1255–63.

6. Wald DS, Bestwick JP, Raiman L, et al. Randomised trial of text messaging on adherence to cardiovascular preventive treatment (INTERACT trial). PLoS One 2014;9(12):e114268.

7. Rifkin DE, Abdelmalek JA, Miracle CM, et al. Linking clinic and home: a randomized, controlled clinical effectiveness trial of real-time, wireless blood pressure monitoring for older patients with kidney disease and hypertension. Blood Press Monit 2013; 18(1):8–15.

8. Aungst T. Apple app store still leads Android in total number of medical apps. MedPage Today 2013. Available at: http://www.imedicalapps.com/2013/07/apple-android-medical-app/. Accessed December 13, 2015.

9. Ritterband LM, Thorndike FP, Gonder-Frederick LA, et al. Efficacy of an Internet-based behavioral intervention for adults with insomnia. Arch Gen Psychiatry 2009;66(7):692–8.

10. Golay A, Girard A, Grandin S, et al. A new educational program for patients suffering from sleep apnea syndrome. Patient Educ Couns 2006;60(2):220–7.

11. Jean Wiese H, Boethel C, Phillips B, et al. CPAP compliance: video education may help! Sleep Med 2005;6(2):171–4.

12. Hoy CJ, Vennelle M, Kingshott RN, et al. Can intensive support improve continuous positive airway pressure use in patients with the sleep apnea/hypopnea syndrome? Am J Respir Crit Care Med 1999; 159(4 Pt 1):1096–100.

13. DeMolles DA, Sparrow D, Gottlieb DJ, et al. A pilot trial of a telecommunications system in sleep apnea management. Med Care 2004;42(8):764–9.

14. Stepnowsky CJ, Palau JJ, Marler MR, et al. Pilot randomized trial of the effect of wireless telemonitoring on compliance and treatment efficacy in obstructive sleep apnea. J Med Internet Res 2007;9(2):e14.

15. Fox N, Hirsch-Allen AJ, Goodfellow E, et al. The impact of a telemedicine monitoring system on positive airway pressure adherence in patients with obstructive sleep apnea: a randomized controlled trial. Sleep 2012;35(4):477–81.

16. Kuna ST, Shuttleworth D, Chi L, et al. Web-based access to positive airway pressure usage with or without an initial financial incentive improves treatment use in patients with obstructive sleep apnea. Sleep 2015;38(8):1229–36.

17. Stepnowsky C, Edwards C, Zamora T, et al. Patient perspective on use of an interactive website for sleep apnea. Int J Telemed Appl 2013;2013: 239382.

18. Hardy W, Powers J, Jasko JG, et al. SleepMapper. A mobile application and website to engage sleep apnea patients in PAP therapy and improve adherence to treatment. Philips White Paper. Available at: http://cdn.sleepreviewmag.com/sleeprev/2014/06/SleepMapper-Adherence-White-Paper.pdf. Accessed January 17, 2016.

19. Munafo D, Hevener W, Crocker M, et al. A telehealth program for CPAP adherence reduces labor and yields similar adherence and efficacy when compared to standard of care. Sleep Breath 2016. [Epub ahead of print].

20. Chang J, Liang J, Hwang D, et al. Impact of interactive web-based education and automated feedback program on CPAP adherence for the treatment of obstructive sleep apnea (Abstract). SLEEP 2016; Denver, CA, 2016.

21. Comstock J. Price Waterhouse: 1 in 5 Americans owns a wearable, 1 in 10 wears them daily. Available at: http://mobihealthnews.com/37543/pwc-1-in-5-americans-owns-a-wearable-1-in-10-wears-them-daily/. Accessed September 11, 2015.

22. Fitness tracker buying guide. Consumer Reports. Available at: http://www.consumerreports.org/cro/fitness-trackers/buying-guide.htm. Accessed December 17, 2015.

23. Kell J. These new wearables aren't for your wrist. Fortunate. Available at: http://fortune.com/2016/01/16/wearables-not-on-your-wrist/. Accessed January 17, 2016.

24. Bhat S, Ferraris A, Gupta D, et al. Is there a clinical role for smartphone sleep apps? Comparison of sleep cycle detection by a smartphone application to polysomnography. J Clin Sleep Med 2015;11(7): 709–15.

25. Prindle D. These sensor-studded headphones can sense when you're in deep sleep, trigger lucid dreams. Yahoo. Available at: https://www.yahoo.com/tech/sensor-studded-headphones-sense-deep-192917652.html. Accessed January 17, 2016.

26. Evenson KR, Goto MM, Furberg RD, et al. Systematic review of the validity and reliability of consumer-wearable activity trackers. Int J Behav Nutr Phys Act 2015;12(1):159.

27. Meltzer LJ, Hiruma LS, Avis K, et al. Comparison of a commercial accelerometer with polysomnography and actigraphy in children and adolescents. Sleep 2015;38(8):1323–30.

28. Lorig K, Ritter PL, Villa FJ, et al. Community-based peer-led diabetes self-management: a randomized trial. Diabetes Educ 2009;35(4):641–51.

29. Parthasarathy S, Wendel C, Haynes PL, et al. A pilot study of CPAP adherence promotion by peer buddies with sleep apnea. J Clin Sleep Med 2013; 9(6):543–50.

30. What is population health management? Wellcentive. Available at: http://www.wellcentive.com/what-is-population-health-management/. Accessed October 1, 2015.

Novel Approaches to the Management of Sleep-Disordered Breathing

 CrossMark

Todd D. Morgan, DMD

KEYWORDS

- Sleep-disordered breathing • Oral appliance • Oropharyngeal exercise • Myofunctional therapy
- Oropharyngeal exercise • Calibration • Dental sleep • Positional therapy

KEY POINTS

- For several reasons, continuous positive airway pressure (CPAP) intolerance is widespread, leading physicians to consider alternative treatments for patients with sleep-disordered breathing.
- Novel treatment options, such as oral appliances, positional therapy, pharmacologic therapy, expiratory positive airway pressure, and myofunctional approaches, are emerging that serve as alternative to nasal CPAP.
- Selection of an appropriate alternative therapy, including newer surgical approaches, oral appliance therapy, positional therapy, and orthodontic therapy, should be made based on an evaluation of each patient's personal needs and a review of their phenotypic traits.

 Video content accompanies this article at http://www.sleep.theclinics.com/

INTRODUCTION

Sleep-disordered breathing (SDB) conditions exist along a continuum of severity, ranging from "benign" snoring on rare occasions to profound collapse of the upper airway, which is associated with significant cardiovascular risk and increased mortality. Obstructive sleep apnea (OSA) is the largest subset of significant SDB presentations and is considered one of the most prevalent medical disorders in developed countries, affecting about 20% of the US population. Benign snoring is ubiquitous, affecting upward of 100 million people in the United States alone. Contrary to being held simply as a social malady, however, loud and chronic snoring has been associated with hypertension, carotid artery disease, and increased motor vehicle crashes, implying a pathologic role.

According to the American Academy of Sleep Medicine (AASM), the first choice of treatment for patients with moderate or severe OSA is continuous positive airway pressure (CPAP).[1] First described in 1981,[2] positive pressure devices work by splinting the airway open to facilitate proper airflow. Manufactured and developed for widespread use during the 1980s and 1990s, traditional CPAP has since undergone many technological advancements that have improved patient satisfaction. Despite this, however, adherence to positive airway pressure (PAP) therapy remains relatively poor, leading providers on a search for alternative treatment options.

Several novel approaches to treating snoring and sleep apnea have emerged that may be better suited for milder SDB. Dental devices, primarily introduced in the 1990s and 2000s, have gained popularity among dentists and sleep physicians primarily for consideration as a "rescue" therapy for those patients intolerant to CPAP. In recent years and as empirical evidence has grown, oral appliance therapy (OAT) has gained momentum

Conflicts of Interest: Intellectual property owner in the Apnea Guard Trial Oral Appliance; Inventor- Pharyngeal Training Appliance.
Oral Medicine, Scripps Memorial Hospital, 320 Santa Fe Drive, Encinitas, CA 92024, USA
E-mail address: todd@toddmorgan.com

sleep.theclinics.com

as a first-line therapy in mild or moderate OSA. Other novel nonsurgical approaches that have demonstrated a positive impact on SDB include expiratory positive airway pressure (EPAP), nasal dilators, oral negative pressure devices, positional therapies, orthodontic expansion, oropharyngeal exercise (OPE)/myofunctional therapies, and pharmacologic therapy.

This article explores the evolving role of newer technology and improvements to therapies that may serve as an alternative to, or work in tandem with, PAP machines that may lead to better adherence, patient satisfaction, and improved public health.

Surgical Treatment Options for Obstructive Sleep Apnea

Surgical procedures are less commonly deployed in the treatment of OSA and usually considered only after conservative modalities have failed. Most clinicians are quite familiar with the array of soft tissue surgeries available to OSA patients, and those are listed in **Box 1**. For purposes of this article, the focus will be narrowed to 2 particular approaches that are recently gaining momentum: a revised version of uvulopalatopharyngoplasty (UPPP) and bariatric surgery.

Bariatric surgery

More than 2 of 3 patients with OSA are obese, making obesity the most important risk factor for OSA.[3] Weight loss, therefore, is an important tool for the sleep physician, who must consider all of the surgical and nonsurgical options available to their patients. In a 5-year observational study by Tuomilehto and colleagues,[4] following 57 patients who used dietary and lifestyle changes to lose weight, the progression of OSA was stalled in all but 2 patients. Most of those who were able to maintain their weight loss (n = 13/20) demonstrated a sustained reduction in Apnea-Hypopnea Index (AHI), which was curative in milder cases. In another study comparing bariatric surgical patients to traditional diet and exercise

---

Box 1
Upper airway soft tissue surgical modalities for treatment of obstructive sleep apnea

Uvulopalatopharyngoplasty

Laser-assisted uvuloplasty

Adenotonsillectomy

Genioglossal advancement

Hyoid suspension

Nasal surgery

---

programs, an even greater weight loss and drop in AHI were seen in the surgical patient group.[5]

Several permutations on techniques used for bariatric surgery are available and all have been shown to assist in significant weight loss, including restrictive surgeries, such as gastric banding that reduces stomach capacity, or resection surgeries, such as gastric bypass. One recent novel approach delivers a rechargeable implanted device to the abdomen that can send intermittent signals of satiations to the brain via the vagus nerve trunk (Maestro EnteroMedics Inc, St. Paul, MN, USA). In a controlled trial of 239 subjects, the implanted device demonstrated a significantly greater weight loss in the active group versus control.[6]

Uvulopalatopharyngoplasty

UPPP was first described as a surgery for OSA by Fujita and colleagues[7] in 1981. Their study of 54 patients who underwent the procedure and then were retested with polysomnography (PSG) about 1 year later experienced a significant drop in their postoperative AHI by almost 50%. Predictors of success were hard to identify, however, and it is interesting that responders to the UPPP showed a highly significant postoperative increase in anterior tongue strength.[7] In 1996, the UPPP procedure was modified by Powell and colleagues[8] to predominantly become a flap procedure, which touted less postoperative pain and was reversible. A recent review of the literature on UPPP outcomes, however, still only demonstrated an overall success rate of 33%, even while using a relaxed definition of success as a drop by 50% in AHI and less than 15 per hour. Despite lackluster results in many patients, UPPP procedures continue to be the most frequently performed surgery for OSA in the United States.[9]

Oral Appliances

In 2015 the AASM and the American Academy of Dental Sleep Medicine (AADSM) jointly commissioned a 7-member task force to develop recommendations based on the quality of the evidence available.[10] A summary of their recommendations is shown in **Table 1**. In addition, the AADSM in 2013 released "Protocol for Oral Appliance Therapy for Sleep Disordered Breathing in Adults: An Update for 2012" that delineates the collaborative roles of the physician and dentist in the delivery and testing for OAT, based on licensure and scope of practice. Part of the dentist's expertise lies in the selection of an appropriate appliance design of which there have been many permutations through the years as technology has advanced. Recent evidence suggests that mandibular

Table 1
A summary of recommendations provided by a joint commission of the American Academy of Sleep Medicine and the American Academy of Dental Sleep Medicine for 2015

Recommendation Statement	Strength of Recommendation	Quality of Evidence	Benefits vs Harms/ Burdens Assessment
The use of oral appliances for treatment of primary snoring in adults			
It is recommended that sleep physicians prescribe oral appliances, rather than no therapy, for adult patients who request treatment of primary snoring (without OSA)	Standard	High	Benefits clearly outweigh harms
The use of oral appliances for treatment of OSA in adults			
When OAT is prescribed by a sleep physician for an adult patient with OSA, it is suggested that a qualified dentist use a custom, titratable appliance over noncustom oral devices	Guideline	Low	Benefits clearly outweigh hams
It is recommended that sleep physicians consider prescription of oral appliances, rather than no treatment, for adult patients with OSA who are intolerant of CPAP therapy or prefer alternate therapy	Standard	Moderate	Benefits clearly outweigh harms
It is suggested that qualified dentists provide oversight—rather than no follow-up—of OAT in adult patients with OSA, to survey for dental-related side effects or occlusal changes and reduce their incidence	Guideline	Low	Benefits clearly outweigh harms
It is suggested that sleep physicians conduct follow-up sleep testing to improve or confirm treatment efficacy, rather than conduct follow-up without sleep testing, for patients fitted with oral appliances	Guideline	Low	Benefits clearly outweigh harms
It is suggested that sleep physicians and qualified dentists instruct adult patients treated with oral appliances for OSA to return for periodic office visits—as opposed to no follow-up—with a qualified dentist and a sleep physician	Guideline	Low	Benefits clearly outweigh harms

advancement has 2 mechanisms of action that increase airway size: in subjects with low AHI, the entire tongue moves forward, and mandibular advancement also produces lateral airway expansion via a direct connection between the lateral walls and the ramus of the mandible.[11]

Tongue-retaining device

Oral appliances were first introduced to Sleep Medicine in the early 1990s when the tongue-retaining device (TRD) made its debut (**Fig. 1**). Originally developed by Drs Charles Samuelson, Rosalind Cartwright, and Michael Alvarez in 1982,[12] the traditional TRD was shown to be quite effective when custom fabricated to match the individual patient's tongue size. Early on, the

inventors used bee's wax to fashion and shape the tongue bulb. Building a modern customized TRD is labor intensive for the dentist, which results in added cost to the patient. In 2002, the TRD was reinvented by an orthodontist, Dr Christopher Robertson, to become the "off-the-shelf" design shown in **Fig. 2**. The Aveo appliance (Ethics International Business and Trade, Inc, Victoria, Canada) comes in 4 sizes (S, M, L, and XL), although a common anecdotal claim is that "90% of folks fit into a medium." To insert the device, the appliance bulb is compressed and the tongue is inserted, with the flange resting against the front teeth or lips. The negative pressure and the salivary adhesion act to secure and displace the tongue into a forward position. Prefabricated

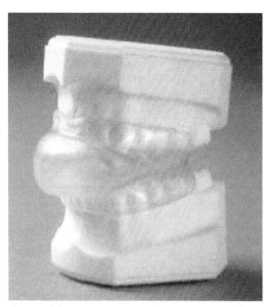

Fig. 1. A laboratory customized TRD. For proper fabrication, a circumferential measurement of the tongue is made with a Kel-gage or floss.

TRDs have made them much easier to prescribe and less expensive for patients, although similar to jaw advancement devices, they have also been shown to produce complications such as bite change.[13]

A novel spin on TRDs is the Winx device (Apnicure, Redwood City, CA, USA). The Winx device works by establishing a vacuum in the oral cavity, which pulls the uvula and soft palate forward and stabilizes the tongue position (**Fig. 3**). In a selected cohort of 63 subjects who tried the Winx device, 20 showed a clinically important response, dropping the mean AHI index by greater than 50%, and lowering Epworth scores from 12.1 to 8.6.[14]

Mandibular repositioning devices

The other class of oral appliances, termed mandibular repositioning devices (MRD), actively

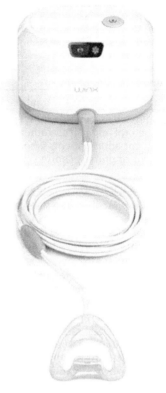

Fig. 3. The Winx device uses negative oral pressure to pull soft tissues forward and secure the tongue. (*Courtesy of* ApniCure, Redwood City, CA; with permission.)

protrudes the mandible and maintains this forward position during sleep (**Fig. 4**). More than 60 design options are now available at last count. Just a few of them include the Herbst, Narval (Res Med), Elastic Mandibular Appliance (Myerson LLC, Chicago, IL, USA), the Thornton Anterior Positioner (Airway Management, Inc, Denton, TX, USA), the Klearway (Great Lakes Orthodontics, Tanawanda, NY, USA) and the Dorsal Fin style appliances (**Fig. 5**). Oral appliances are small, transportable,

Fig. 2. The insertion technique for an off-the-shelf TRD is shown. (*Courtesy of* Glidewell Laboratories, Newport Beach, CA; with permission.)

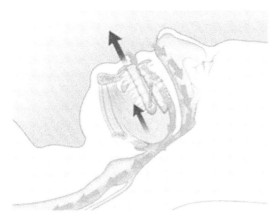

Fig. 4. Oral appliances work by advancing and stabilizing the mandible, which in turn acts to advance the tongue and soft palate, improving airway caliber through a complex interaction among pharyngeal muscles.

but more expensive than CPAP at the beginning of therapy. After the first 2 years of use, however, costs become comparable to CPAP, which requires resupply of components. Side effects to a patient's teeth or bite relationship while using OAT long term are of concern. In a recent review of these side effects, however, researchers determined that although dental changes are common, they are well tolerated overall and seldom

debilitating enough to require discontinuation of therapy in light of their benefit.[15] Dental changes can be mitigated when patients adhere to prescribed repositioning exercises or wear occlusal indexes for a short time in the morning.

Design selection of mandibular repositioning devices

Selection of a specific appliance design by the treating dentist is chiefly dependent on their training and experience in Dental Sleep Medicine (DSM). Other considerations can be made for laboratory processing costs, convenience, durability, ease of adjustability, and even patient preferences that may often be primarily driven by manufacturers' claims made through Internet marketing. A recent study by Almeida and colleagues[16] demonstrated that comfort should be strongly considered if a goal of therapy is long-term adherence. More recent evidence suggests that design selection may impact outcomes in patients with positional OSA. Cistulli and colleagues[17] recently published results from their investigation on positional OSA that showed no important added benefit to using MRD in supine-related OSA. The investigators suggested that design selection may have had an impact on their results because their findings run contrary to previous studies that did show stronger responses in positional

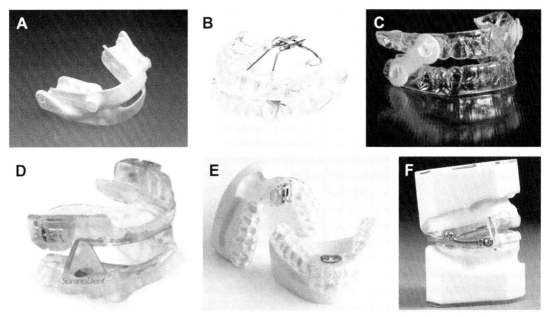

Fig. 5. Several examples of oral appliances are shown that use a variety of materials and hardware that allow for calibration. From top left clockwise: (*A*) Narval, (*B*) Klearway, (*C*) Elastomeric Mandibular Advancement, (*D*) Somnodent, (*E*) Thornton Anterior Positioner (TAP), (*F*) Herbst. (*Courtesy of* [A] ResMed, San Diego, CA, with permission; [B, F] Great Lakes Orthodontics, Tanawanda, NY, with permission; [C] Myerson LLC, Chicago, IL, with permission; [D] SomnoMed, Inc, Frisco, TX, with permission; [E] Glidewell Laboratories, Newport Beach, CA, with permission.)

OSA when a design was selected that prevented the jaw from falling open while supine.[18]

Oral Appliance Calibration Technology

In sleep medicine, the word titration refers to the incremental increase in air pressure, whereas the CPAP mask is worn during laboratory PSG. Similarly, most mandibular advancement devices are designed to accommodate small increases in jaw protrusion, termed "calibration," in order to achieve therapeutic effects and improved management of SDB events. Depending on the patient's chief complaints associated with their OSA, resolution of symptoms, such as snoring, waking headache, frequency of awakenings, and fatigue (due to sleep fragmentation), may improve while calibration progresses. Home sleep testing (HST) provides the DSM practitioner with an objective means to measure successful positioning of the mandible in both the protrusive and the vertical planes. Using HST to "dial in" the best jaw position is an advanced skill in DSM and does not replace diagnostic or definitive follow-up sleep testing by the physician.

Several investigations have illustrated the influence that subtle protrusive adjustments of an oral appliance can have on SDB outcomes,[19–21] with one group reporting adjustments as small as 0.25 mm improving snoring intensity and respiratory disturbance index.[22] Calibration of an oral appliance can take place in either the protrusive or the vertical dimension, as illustrated in **Fig. 6**. The precise influence of added vertical opening within the scheme of the final jaw position is not well understood, but there seems to be a role when taking gender and tongue size into account.[23]

Multiple sleep testing titration

A combination of sleep testing modalities can be used to "dial in" the correct jaw position for OAT. In one 2011 study at Walter Reed Hospital, Holley and colleagues demonstrated in a group of 497 soldiers that using a combination of strategies for final jaw positioning was helpful.[24] By using a sequence of patient subjective reporting, followed by repeated HST, followed then by a final PSG, outcomes were improved in the group by 33% when compared with HST alone. Similar results were also found in another study by Almeida and Parker,[25] where they added a final titration protocol during PSG that ordered the attending technician to awaken the patient sequentially to further advance the jaw while recording changes in AHI during epochs of time in that position (**Fig. 7**). **Fig. 8** shows an example

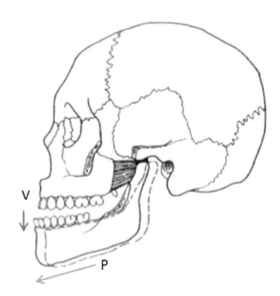

Fig. 6. The diagram illustrates the 2 components of jaw repositioning: (P) protrusion and (V) vertical dimension. Oral appliances combine these principles to different degrees to improve outcomes. Some degree of vertical opening automatically accompanies protrusion due to the dynamic arc of TMJ translation.

of one such strategy for OAT titration in the laboratory.

Predictive jaw positioning: real-time sleep testing

One unique method uses a remotely controlled servo motor device attached to a dentist-generated oral tray system (Matrix-Zepher, Inc). In the laboratory setting, a technologist remotely adds small increments of jaw protrusion based on real-time polysomnographic study readings. In a further advancement of this technology, HST is used in place of PSG, and the same servo actuator moves the lower jaw forward sequentially based on an algorithm derived from the monitor's oximetry and nasal flow cannula data. The goal of this technique is to provide the DSM practitioner with an accurate target for final starting jaw protrusive positioning for the customized MRD.[26]

Predicting starting jaw position: measurement-based

Although titration strategies are becoming more refined, the starting position of the mandible is critical in that relief from SDB can be facilitated very early in the therapy. In another validated technique that uses a trial oral appliance to determine correct starting position for a custom MRD, the technician or dentist uses a system that can predict the correct protrusive and vertical position of the jaw

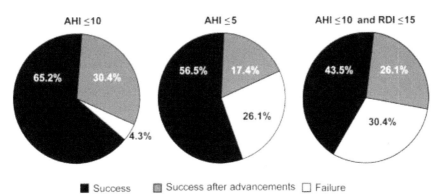

Fig. 7. The added benefit of overnight sequential titration of an oral appliance during PSG. Depending on the definition of success, up to 90% of subjects treated turned out well. (*Courtesy of* F. Almeida, DDS, MSc, PhD, Vancouver, BC.)

Protocol for MRD Titration
In a Sleep Lab

The patient presenting tonight for PSG has been wearing the oral appliance for at least three weeks. He/she has self-adjusted the appliance to a starting treatment position (STP). The Technician is responsible for waking the patient as described below and **having them self-adjust their device in order to optimize treatment.**

The dentist and patient have <u>usually</u> tested the patient's comfort level with additional titration prior to the overnight.   However, should the patient state that any further titration is painful, end further titration/advancement.

Technique:

1.   Evaluate the patient at the TP for at least the first 1.5 hours or until the first REM period. If AHI >10 supine then wake patient and make one forward adjustment (adjustment depends on type of appliance design, but instruct the patient to make "one standard adjustment forward"
2.   Evaluate the patient for the next 1–2hrs, observing REM and supine if possible. Make an additional adjustment as needed to reduce AHI to <10.
3.   Repeat number (2) for each new time segment until study completion.
4.   Record any side effects at titration end-point_____

5.   Record the following parameter at each of the treatment positions:

	Starting Tx Position (STP)	1ˢᵗ Adjustment	2ⁿᵈ Adjustment	3ʳᵈ Adjustment
RDI				
RDI supine				
Mean Q2				
Time<90%				
Lowest saturation				
Snoring Index				
Inspiratory flow Limitation				

Number of alcoholic drinks tonight_____ Medications taken tonight_____

_____

Technician: _____ Date:_____

Patient Name/DOB:_____ Phone:_____

Fig. 8. One example is given for a laboratory PSG-driven protocol for final calibration of an oral appliance. Given that different device designs use differing adjustment mechanisms, the patient, not the technician, makes their "familiar" adjustment when awakened and instructed to do so. A minimal impact on sleep efficiency has been observed. (*Courtesy of* Dr Todd D. Morgan, DMD, Encinitas, CA; with permission.)

through a proprietary algorithm (Apnea Guard; Advance Brain Monitoring, Carlsbad, CA, USA). This system has the added benefit of providing the patient with immediate treatment of their SDB while waiting the weeks necessary for dental laboratory fabrication (**Fig. 9**). Based on a validation study demonstrating outcome equivalency between the Apnea Guard and custom appliances,[27] the device can provide the sleep physician an opportunity to identify responders to OAT by wearing the device during an overnight test before oral appliance fabrication.

Oral Appliance Adherence Monitoring Technology

Menn and colleagues[28] in 1996 were first to report patient adherence to using a "jaw advancement device." Of those 20 subjects available for telephone follow-up, 70% stated they were still using the device nightly after 3.4 years. Whereas previous studies on oral appliance adherence depended on patient report and wear-time logs much like CPAP before electronically generated compliance, emerging electronic technology will now allow for adherence monitoring of oral appliances, using an embedded electronic sensor that provides the readout (**Fig. 10**).

In a recent 3-month prospective study using new electronic monitoring of adherence to oral appliance use by data download, Vanderveken and colleagues[29] showed adherence to be 6.6 ± 1.3 hours of use per night. In his cohort, 84% were termed "regular users" as defined by at least 4 hours of use per night, the same definition of

adequate adherence applied to PAP therapy. In this context and this group of subjects then, adherence to OAT is markedly superior to CPAP. Several manufacturers of adherence sensors are presently under US Food and Drug Administration (FDA) scrutiny at the time of this publication, and the FDA requires that each sensor manufacturer must submit for clearance for each given oral appliance design. Thus far, only the DentiTrac device (Braebon Medical, Kanata, ON) has been approved for clinical use in the United States. The DrentiTrac sensor measures time worn based on temperature sampling as often as 1-second intervals, and a built-in accelerometer that captures "true" wear-time by temperature and movement. Battery life depends on sampling rate.

Noncustom Oral Appliances

Prefabricated or so-called, boil-and-bite oral devices, have been widely advertised through the Internet for the treatment of snoring and even OSA. Previous studies have described several problems associated with prefabricated designs, such as increased bulk and tendency for tooth movement or bite complications, also showing reduced efficacy and satisfaction.[30] In addition, despite some newer designs that incorporate adjustability aspects, true control over a measured jaw advancement position is not possible as in customized devices. Although the literature does not support their use in replacement of custom OAT, prefabricated devices may have a role in determining a subjective response to jaw advancement maneuvers. Given the lack of robust predictors of response to OAT, the sleep physician may find utility in determining response through a trial of an over-the-counter device.

Positional Therapy

Traditionally, the folksy recommendation to patients with positional obstructive sleep apnea (POSA) has been very simple: sew tennis balls to the back of a nightshirt. However, this approach was found to be too uncomfortable by most patients to be effective.[31] Alternatively, the use of padding, foam, and even air bladders worn around the waist may be more comfortable, and effective, in reducing a patient's time spent supine and their overall sleep apnea. Two examples of these products are shown in **Fig. 11**.

Typically, positional therapies have been largely overlooked as a stand-alone therapy for OSA, but the AASM Clinical Guidelines do recognize/recommend positional therapy as an alternative to CPAP in POSA in patients who have CPAP intolerance.[32,33] POSA is defined as a patient having a

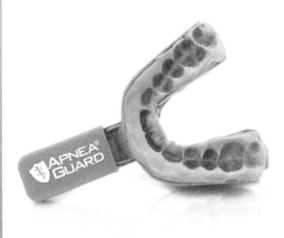

Fig. 9. The Apnea Guard trial device. (*Courtesy of* Advanced Brain Monitoring, Inc., Carlsbad, CA; with permission.)

A

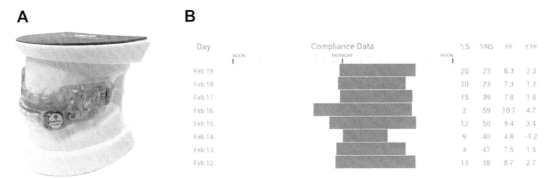

B

Day	Compliance Data	%S	%NS	Hr	± Hr
	NOON MIDNIGHT NOON				
Feb 19		20	23	8.3	2.3
Feb 18		20	23	7.3	1.3
Feb 17		15	39	7.8	1.8
Feb 16		2	59	10.7	4.7
Feb 15		12	50	9.4	3.4
Feb 14		9	40	4.8	-1.2
Feb 13		4	47	7.5	1.5
Feb 12		13	38	8.7	2.7

Fig. 10. (*A, B*) New technology will now allow for electronic tracking of oral appliance adherence. The nickel-sized chip is embedded within the appliance acrylic. A typical readout combines time worn (temperature sampling plus motion detection). (*Courtesy of* Braebon Medical, Kanata, ON; with permission.)

supine AHI severity 2 times greater than the non-supine AHI.[34] Previous reports estimate that 55% of patients diagnosed with SDB have POSA. However, more recently, it has been reported that as many as 70% of patients with an AHI less than 60 events per hour have a positional component to their disease.[34] Asian populations are thought to be at an even greater risk for POSA due to distinctive craniofacial form.[35]

Three novel approaches to positional therapy are shown in **Fig. 12**. Two of them deploy vibrotactile (similar to a cell phone) technology, which delivers a biofeedback signal to the neck or chest when a patient assumes the supine position. The third uses an audio recording (either the patient or their bed partner) that plays through ear buds to the patient, reminding them to go to their side. Both of the vibrotactile devices have been found to be effective in improving sleep quality and reducing the overall number of arousals per hour.[36,37] Furthermore, after 30 nights of use, complaints of daytime drowsiness, depression, and insomnia were improved. One developer

(Night Shift; Advanced Brain Monitoring, Carlsbad, CA, USA) demonstrated that across 30 nights of use, user compliance exceeded 90%.

Expiratory Positive Airway Pressure

EPAP is a nasal device that consists of disposable adhesive devices that are placed over the nostrils and provide resistance to flow by virtue of a mechanical valve. Specifically, EPAP is designed to provide high resistance to flow during exhalation, but low resistance to flow during inhalation (**Fig. 13**). The high expiratory resistance provides pneumatic splinting and makes the upper airway more resistant to collapse on subsequent inspiration. In a 3-month multicenter clinical trial, nasal EPAP was shown to be clinically helpful in improving the AHI, O_2 nadir, and sleep quality. Subjects reported that they were able to wear EPAP all night for approximately 88% of nights and side effects were mild.[38] The investigators reported there were some clinical difficulties with the proper nightly application of the EPAP, but the

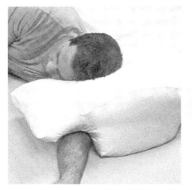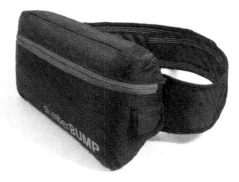

Fig. 11. One example of a foam-filled belt and an "anti-snore" pillow designed to prevent/reduce time spent supine during sleep. (*Courtesy of* Snorestore, Harow, United Kingdom; with permission.)

A 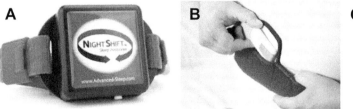 B C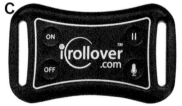

Fig. 12. (*A–C*) Three positional training devices that are marketed to discourage supine sleep that are either worn around the neck or chest. Two use an accelerometer that triggers a vibrational signal; one uses a recorded voice command. (*Courtesy of* [A] Advanced Brain Monitoring, Inc, Carlsbad, CA; with permission; [B] NightBalance B.V., Molengraaffsingel 12-14 2629 JD, Delft, The Netherlands; with permission; and [C] Snoremart, Belleview, Washington; with permission.)

effectiveness of EPAP in this study compares favorably to other treatment modalities.

Pharmacologic Treatment of Obstructive Sleep Apnea

Pharmacologic treatment of SDB is by no means a new concept because drugs like oxygen and acetazolamide demonstrated early on a benefit to selected patients with OSA.[39] However, pharmacologic therapies have not gained widespread consideration due to a lack of controlled trial and the ready access to devices and surgery. Given the reluctance patients to use CPAP and the increasing demand patients have for more options, the divergence away from this "one-size-fits-all" paradigm is explicable.

One emerging pharmacologic model, developed by David White and colleagues,[40] fits very well into this individualized approach to the treatment of SDB. In short, based on the individual's physiologic traits, a variety of drug therapies may be deployed that can influence and have measureable effects on sleep systems, such as arousal threshold, upper airway muscle response to a threat, and loop gain.

It is thought that there is a wide variability in the level of respiratory drive required to awaken a patient with an OSA, and that perhaps one-third of these patients have a low arousal threshold.[41] Elevating this threshold, therefore, may bring a meaningful therapeutic benefit. In one example of this model, it may be possible to improve a given patient's OSA by manipulation of their arousal threshold using hypnotics. Eckert and Younes[42] have shown that in their subjects with OSA, arousability from a respiratory challenge can be quite variable and may be dependent on a tolerated level of epiglottal respiratory pressure. They further showed that by giving a hypnotic drug like trazadone or eszopiclone, higher epiglottal (closing) pressures could be tolerated before arousal occurred in these subjects and, in turn, reduced AHI.

Predictive Models for Selecting Alternative Therapies

CPAP is regarded as the gold standard of treatment for OSA, as suggested by the published AASM Standards of Practice Protocols.[32] The universal efficacy of positive pressure devices is

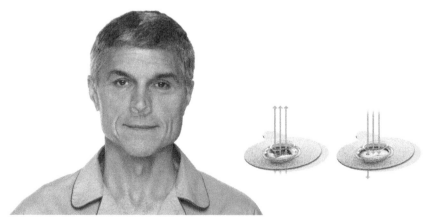

Fig. 13. Nasal EPAP device. Single-use valves are inserted over each nostril and sealed with an adhesive backing. (*Courtesy of* Provent Sleep Therapy, LLC, Manchester, NH; with permission.)

easily understood by the pneumatic splinting of the upper airway, regardless of any potentially disabled airway dilator muscle defense response. Jordan and colleagues[43] have shown that inadequate muscle responses in SDB may constitute an important component of airway collapse.

Phenotyping models: oral appliance therapy

Previously, it had been difficult to predict response to OAT. However, progress has been made by some researchers recently that is helping to develop predictive models that use information from the sleep study as well as morphometric traits. Earlier work has previously identified predictors for OAT response that include traits such as younger age, less obesity, a lower body mass index (BMI), and female gender. Some of these predictors have been consistently supported by others and some refuted. A recent study by Cistulli and colleagues[17] of 425 patients explored in detail some of the anthropomorphic details from PSG generated sleep data that may aid in identifying responders to OAT. The group found that younger age, lower BMI, lower neck circumference, and lower baseline BMI remain strong predictors. In terms of sleep study findings, they reported that efficacy was also related to sleep stage, showing that OAT had only a 12% response rate during rapid eye movement sleep. Intersecting with any predictive model for OAT is determining the correct selection of design, which remains more of an art than a science.

The role of pharyngeal muscle response

Most treatment modalities besides CPAP depend to some degree on an intact and appropriate muscle response, which could be lacking in certain patient phenotypes. This difference may explain to a large extent the incomplete responses to surgery and OAT, for example, and may in a larger sense restrict a clinician's viewpoint toward emerging therapies and technology. Uncertainty surrounding individual response to OAT has been one roadblock to dental devices developing widespread use. When the variable response of pharyngeal muscles to a challenge is afforded, one can begin to explain OAT failures, and also when unexpected favorable responses are observed and may also be why cone beam computed tomography (CBCT) and MRI imaging studies have fallen short of helping to predict response because the true "muscles are sleeping" airway is not being viewed.

As mentioned above, the technique of drug-induced sleep endoscopy (DISE) may theoretically facilitate a view of how sleeping upper airway muscles behave as well as the site of collapse along the length of the pharynx. Recent studies using DISE have demonstrated that certain pharyngeal opening patterns with jaw advancement may predict a positive outcome with OAT.[44] In addition, because the jaw can be advanced in real-time during DISE while an oral appliance is in place, the opportunity also presents to "customize" the jaw protrusive position to be concurrent to the most ideal opening (Video 1).

Oral Myofunctional Therapy

SDB, like any chronic disease process, develops in a multifactorial manner, with anatomic and pharyngeal muscle responses at the forefront. Upper airway dilator muscles are crucial to the maintenance of pharyngeal patency, and emerging evidence exists that these muscle have diminished responses over time.[43]

In a broad sense, oral myofunctional therapy refers to either the retraining of oral and pharyngeal muscle or the strengthening of these muscles with the goal of correcting abnormal or inadequate function. The oral myofunctional therapist aims to correct muscle function by retraining tongue and lip position to their proper orientation, while also using oral strength training to a reinforce desired changes in swallowing pattern. This training alone has been shown to improve SDB in several recent studies. In a systematic review of 9 studies and a total of 120 patients,[45] Camacho and colleagues[45] demonstrated positive outcomes in several sleep parameters. As a whole, the collective AHI dropped by approximately 50% in these groups. Oxygen nadir and snoring improved significantly as well. The overall drop in Epworth scores went from 14.8 to 8.2.

OPE alone has also been shown in the past to improve SDB, although the overlap with traditional myofunctional training and the impact of concomitant repositioning of the tongue and lips while performing OPE need to be considered. The exact mechanism of action on muscles while playing an instrument like the didgeridoo, a bassoon, or an oboe are not understood, but all 3 of these instruments require a skill known as "circular breathing" to play well. Singing, even nonprofessionally, has been shown to improve snoring.[46] Several noncontrolled studies have been done that have demonstrated improvements in OSA with exercise, and those studies have led to further investigation. In a 2009 OPE study by Guimarães and colleagues[47] of—Brazilian men with moderate OSA, significant improvements were seen in AHI and other measures, such as daytime sleepiness and sleep quality when a specific regiment of isometric and isotonic exercises derived from speech therapy were used in the active group of 10 men. Eight men displayed a shift from moderate to mild OSA, while 2 men had a complete response with no residual OSA.

Many patients are very interested in self-help approaches to their health care and are looking for natural solutions. Studies are currently underway that will aim to show the utility of OPE as stand-alone therapy or as an adjunctive therapy that may improve OAT outcomes (Dr Malhotra, personal communication, 2016).

Orthodontics

The age-old adage "form follows function" was coined by an American architect named Louis Sullivan and means that the shape of a building or object should be predicated by or based on its intended function or purpose. In biology, this saying has been interpreted to mean that the functional aspects of a biological system drive the shape of structures (bone) to that function. In the presence of inadequate or abnormal muscle function, it would be expected that structures adapt (obey) those improper functions. One example of this is the presence of a tongue-thrust swallowing pattern driving a change in the shape of facial bones or the position of teeth (**Fig. 14**).

Concepts regarding "long faces" are well accepted in orthodontics because these processes are primarily responsible for loss of dental arch width and subsequent malocclusion.[48] From the standpoint of SDB, these phenotypic traits also place these patients at greater risk for SDB due to a concurrently reduced upper airway volume[49] Cistulli and colleagues[50] have previously demonstrated the prevalence of OSA is linked to certain phenotypic (narrow) facial shapes as well as the utility of corrective surgically assisted maxillary expansion and orthodontics in men with OSA. In their study of 8 men and 2 women with moderate OSA, a reduction in SDB of more than 50% was seen.[51]

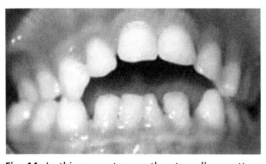

Fig. 14. In this case a tongue-thrust swallow pattern has driven the open bite relationship seen in this 5 year old. This swallow pattern will likely persist into adulthood, setting the stage for malocclusion and OSA. (*Courtesy of* Dr Todd D. Morgan, Encinitas, CA; with permission.)

Orthodontic approaches to correction of these types of malocclusions have for the most part largely ignored the impaired function of the upper airway that is often associated. The pediatric sleep literature is rich with evidence that maxillary expansion is often curative of SDB in children, but would a similar approach be appropriate in adults? Although the capability of bony expansion of facial bones in adults is controversial within the orthodontic field, recent work by Singh and colleagues[52] has shown promising results with adult nonsurgical expansion in treating SDB. Their work is conceptually based on the epigenetic premise that the potential for ideal growth and development of the craniofacial system remains intact within an individual and that renewed bony growth can be unleashed and accomplished with expansion type oral appliances. In a recent study, Singh and colleagues[52] demonstrated in 10 consecutive adult patients that their expansion device technology gradually improved the AHI scores in these subjects over 8.7 months time by 65.9%. The improvement in SDB is attributable to the remodeling of the midfacial bones and the upper airway in these subjects, which was demonstrated on CBCT scanning (**Fig. 15**). Furthermore, in these trials, this method expansion for the treatment of SDB has been shown to be successful regardless of age or gender.

Combination Therapy

Combining therapies when one approach falls short of a desired outcome is highly logical, because most therapies are not mutually exclusive and often complement each other. However, a significant move in this direction has not occurred because the traditional referral process encourages the paradigm of simply moving a patient from one modality to the next. Some progress has been made, however, in the practice of combining OAT with PAP therapy. Because one of the major complaints from patients about PAP therapy is the mask interface, leaks, and discomfort from tight straps, it is encouraging to see reports emerging that demonstrate wearing an oral appliance conjointly with PAP can lower required pressures. El-Solh and colleagues[53] showed in one recent study that combining OAT with APAP effectively lowered treatment pressure in 10 patients by an average of 2 cmH$_2$O and improved the mean oxygen nadir. Together, the combination of PAP with OAT was superior in all respects to outcomes with either treatment alone. It should be further noted that from a clinical aspect, many practitioners have found anecdotally that combining OAT with PAP can remedy mouth leaks

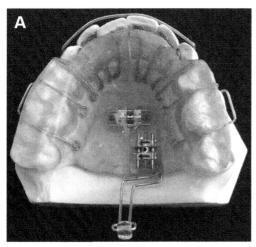
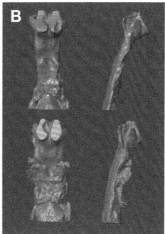

Fig. 15. The DNA appliance is a novel orthodontic device designed to expand the maxilla and therefore the upper airway dimensions at any age (*A*). In adults with OSA, changes in the upper airway are evident with CBCT scanning (*B*). (*Courtesy of* G. Dave Singh DDSc, PhD, DMD, BioModeling Solutions, Inc, Beaverton, OR; with permission.)

and facilitate full face mask seal, presumably by stabilizing the mandible.

Several products have been developed that fully connect a mask interface with an intraoral appliance, eliminating the need for straps altogether. One such device (TAP PAP; Airway Management, Inc) is shown in **Fig. 16**. In this type of interface, a nasal pillow mask is anchored to the maxilla (bone) via the dentition and is fully customized to fit the teeth by the dentist. Mask seal is claimed to be superior because the nasal pillows are held ridged and slippage is averted.

SUMMARY

The novel treatment options that are becoming available to sleep medicine practitioners continue to expand. New treatment approaches are often a product of developing more fully the understanding of the pathophysiology involved with SDB, or are developed as technological advances in existing therapies. Some of the most important improvements have come with the development of PAP technology. Improved mask interfaces that have not been discussed here, but the reader is urged to explore this on their own.

Future research and technology hold promise for more answers to the call for novel SDB treatments as the health care costs associated with untreated OSA burgeons. PAP therapy remains at the forefront for the treatment of SDB, but when the spectrum of severity of SDB and adherence to CPAP is considered, the sleep medicine practitioner is compelled to consider other options available for milder cases. Patients too are driving a trend that is leading toward a more tailored approach to care as they become savvy to the variety of treatment planning options.

Too often, however, alternative treatments fall short of desired outcomes either by measure of the definition of success or due to failed adherence to therapy. Certainly, relaxing the expectations of

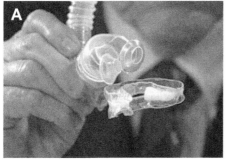
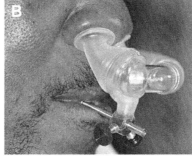

Fig. 16. Combining PAP with an oral appliance interface eliminates the need for head straps and achieves a superior seal allowing therapeutic pressure reduction. (*Courtesy of* Airway Management, Inc, Carrollton, TX; with permission.)

outcomes based on traditional metrics of a final AHI less than 5 is worth considering, especially when quality-of-life treatment goals and patient satisfaction are achieved. Perhaps future studies should focus on combining therapies that complement each other, encourage collaboration among specialties, and move patients closer to the desired goals.

SUPPLEMENTARY DATA

Supplementary data related to this article can be found online at http://dx.doi.org/10.1016/j.jsmc.2016.03.001.

REFERENCES

1. Kushida CA, Chediak A, Berry RB, et al. Clinical guidelines for the manual titration of positive airway pressure in patients with obstructive sleep apnea. J Clin Sleep Med 2008;4(2):157–71.
2. Sullivan CE, Issa FG, Berthon-Jones M, et al. Reversal of obstructive sleep apnoea by continuous positive airway pressure applied through the nares. Lancet 1981;1(8225):862–5.
3. Young T, Shatrud J, Peppard PE. Risk factors for obstructive sleep apnea in adults. JAMA 2004;291: 2013–6.
4. Tuomilehto H, Seppa J, Usityupa M. The impact of weight reduction in the prevention of progression of obstructive sleep apnea: an explanatory analysis of a five year observational follow-up trial. Sleep Med 2014;15:329–35.
5. Ashrafian H, Toma T, Rowland SP, et al. Bariatric surgery or non-surgical weight loss for obstructive sleep apnoea? A systematic review and comparison of meta-analyses. Obes Surg 2015;25(7):1239–50.
6. Ikramuddin S, Blackstone R, Brancatisano A, et al. Effect of reversible intermittent intra-abdominal vagal nerve blockade on morbid obesity: the recharge clinical trial. JAMA 2014;312(9):915–22.
7. Fujita S, Conway W, Zorick F, et al. Surgical correction of anatomic abnormalities in obstructive sleep apnea syndrome: uvulopalatopharyngoplasty. Otolaryngol Head Neck Surg 1981;89(6):923–34.
8. Powell N, Riley R, Guilleminault C, et al. A reversible uvulopalatal flap for snoring and sleep apnea syndrome. Sleep 1996;19(7):593–9.
9. Aurora RN, Casey KR, Kristo D, et al, American Academy of Sleep Medicine. Practice parameters for the surgical modifications of the upper airway for obstructive sleep apnea in adults. Sleep 2010; 33(10):1408–13.
10. Ramar K, Dort LC, Katz SG, et al. Clinical practice guideline for the treatment of obstructive sleep apnea and snoring with oral appliance therapy: an update for 2015. J Clin Sleep Med 2015;11(7): 773–827.
11. Brown EC, Cheng S, McKenzie DK, et al. Tongue and lateral upper airway movement with mandibular advancement. Sleep 2013;36(3):397–404.
12. Samelson CF. The role of tongue retaining device in treatment of snoring and obstructive sleep apnea. CDS Rev 1988;81(9):44–7.
13. Chen H, Lowe AA, Strauss AM, et al. Dental changes evaluated with a 3D computer-assisted model analysis after long-term tongue retaining device wear in OSA patients. Sleep Breath 2008;12(2):169–78.
14. Colrain IM, Black J, Siegel LC, et al. A multicenter evaluation of oral pressure therapy for the treatment of obstructive sleep apnea. Sleep Med 2013;14(9): 830–7.
15. Doff MH, Finnema KJ, Hoekema A, et al. Long-term oral appliance therapy in obstructive sleep apnea syndrome: a controlled study on dental side effects. Clin Oral Investig 2013;17(2):475–82.
16. Almeida FR, Henrich N, Marra C, et al. Patient preferences and experiences of CPAP and oral appliances for the treatment of obstructive sleep apnea: a qualitative analysis. Sleep Breath 2013;17(2):659–66.
17. Sutherland K, Takaya H, Qian J, et al. Oral appliance treatment response and polysomnographic phenotypes of obstructive sleep apnea. J Clin Sleep Med 2015;11(8):861–8.
18. Chung JW, Enciso R, Levendowski DJ, et al. Patients with positional versus nonpositional obstructive sleep apnea: a retrospective study of risk factors associated with apnea-hypopnea severity. Oral Surg Oral Med Oral Pathol Oral Radiol Endod 2010;110(5): 605–10.
19. Fleury B, Rakotonanahary D, Petelle B, et al. Mandibular advancement titration for obstructive sleep apnea: optimization of the procedure by combining clinical and oximetric parameters. Chest 2004;125(5):1761–7.
20. Kato J, Isono S, Tanaka A, et al. Dose-dependent effects of mandibular advancement on pharyngeal mechanics and nocturnal oxygenation in patients with sleep-disordered breathing. Chest 2000;117(4): 1065–72.
21. Gindre L, Gagnadoux F, Meslier N, et al. Mandibular advancement for obstructive sleep apnea: dose effect on apnea, long-term use and tolerance. Respiration 2008;76(4):386–92.
22. Levendowski DL, Popovic D, Morgan T, et al. Assessment of incremental titration of an oral appliance using home sleep testing: a case study. Presented AADSM conference. Seattle, WA, June 5–7, 2009.
23. Levendowski DL, Popovic D, Morgan T, et al. Assessing change in the apnea/hypopnea index resulting from increased vertical dimension of occlusion of mandibular repositioning devices. Presented AADSM conference. Seattle, WA, June 5–7, 2009.

24. Lettieri CJ, Paolino N, Eliasson AH, et al. Comparison of adjustable and fixed oral appliances for the treatment of obstructive sleep apnea. J Clin Sleep Med 2011;7(5):439–45.

25. Holley AB, Lettieri CJ, Shah AA. Efficacy of an adjustable oral appliance and comparison with continuous positive airway pressure for the treatment of obstructive sleep apnea syndrome. Chest 2011;140(6):1511–6.

26. Remmers J, Charkhandeh S, Grosse J, et al. Remotely controlled mandibular protrusion during sleep predicts therapeutic success with oral appliances in patients with obstructive sleep apnea. Sleep 2013;36(10):1517–25, 1525A.

27. Levendowski D, Morgan T, Westbrook P. Initial evaluation of a titration appliance for temporary treatment of obstructive sleep apnea. J Sleep Disord Ther 2012;1(1). Available at: http://www.omicsgroup.org/journals/sleep-disorders-therapy.php. Accessed April 18, 2016.

28. Menn SJ, Loube DI, Morgan TD, et al. The mandibular repositioning device: role in the treatment of obstructive sleep apnea. Sleep 1996;19(10):794–800.

29. Vanderveken OM, Dieltjens M, Wouters K, et al. Objective measurement of compliance during oral appliance therapy for sleep-disordered breathing. Thorax 2013;68(1):91–6.

30. Tsuda H, Almeida FR, Masumi S, et al. Side effects of boil and bite type oral appliance therapy in sleep apnea patients. Sleep Breath 2010;14(3):227–32.

31. Bignold JJ, Deans-Costi G, Goldsworthy MR, et al. Poor long-term patient compliance with the tennis ball technique for treating positional obstructive sleep apnea. J Clin Sleep Med 2009;5:428–30.

32. Epstein LJ, Kristo D, stroll PJ, et al. Clinical guideline for the evaluation, management and long-term care of obstructive sleep apnea in adults. J Clin Sleep Med 2009;5(3):263–76.

33. Ravesloot MJL, van Maanen JP, Dun L, et al. The undervalued potential of position therapy in position-dependent snoring and obstructive sleep apnea-a review of the literature. Sleep Breath 2013;17(1):3949.

34. Oksenberg AS. Positional therapy for sleep apnea: a promising behavioral therapeutic option still waiting for qualified studies. Sleep Med Rev 2014;18:3–5.

35. Sutherland K, Lee RW, Cistulli PA. Obesity and craniofacial structure as risk factors for obstructive sleep apnoea: impact of ethnicity. Respirology 2012;17:213–22.

36. Van Maanen JP, Meester KA, Dun LN, et al. The sleep position trainer: a new treatment for positional obstructive sleep apnea. Sleep Breath 2013;17(2):771–9.

37. Levendowski DJ, Seagraves S, Popovic D, et al. Assessment of a neck-based treatment and monitoring device for positional obstructive sleep apnea. J Clin Sleep Med 2014;10(8):863–71.

38. Samuel J, Traylor J, Marcus CL. Pilot study of nasal expiratory positive airway pressure devices for the treatment of childhood obstructive sleep apnea syndrome. J Clin Sleep Med 2014;10:663.

39. Chauncey J, Aldrich M. Preliminary findings in the treatment of obstructive sleep apnea with transtracheal oxygen. Sleep 1990;13:167–74.

40. White DP. New therapies for obstructive sleep apnea. Semin Respir Crit Care Med 2014;35(5):621–8.

41. Eckert DJ, White DP, Jordan AS, et al. Defining phenotypic causes of obstructive sleep apnea. Identification of novel therapeutic targets. Am J Respir Crit Care Med 2013;188:996–1004.

42. Eckert DJ, Younes MK. Arousal from sleep: implications for obstructive sleep apnea pathogenesis and treatment. J Appl Physiol 2014;116:302–13.

43. Jordan AS, McSharry DG, Malhotra A. Adult obstructive sleep apnoea. Lancet 2014;383:736.

44. Kent DT, Rogers R, Soose RJ. Drug-induced sedation endoscopy in the evaluation of osa patients with incomplete oral appliance therapy response. Otolaryngol Head Neck Surg 2015;153(2):302–7.

45. Camacho M, Certal V, Abdullatif J, et al. Myofunctional therapy to treat obstructive sleep apnea: a systematic review and meta-analysis. Sleep 2015;38(5):669–75.

46. Pai I, Lo S, Wolf D, et al. The effect of singing on snoring and daytime somnolence. Sleep Breath 2008;12(3):265–8.

47. Guimarães KC, Drager LF, Genta PR, et al. Effects of oropharyngeal exercises on patients with moderate obstructive sleep apnea syndrome. Am J Respir Crit Care Med 2009;179(10):962–6.

48. Cole P. Doctors and dentists: review of a symposium. J Otolaryngol 1989;18(4):135–6.

49. Wang MF, Otsuka T, Akimoto S, et al. Vertical facial height and its correlation with facial width and depth: three dimensional cone beam computed tomography evaluation based on dry skulls. Int J Stomatol Occlusion Med 2013;6:120–9.

50. Lee RW, Sutherland K, Chan AS, et al. Relationship between surface facial dimensions and upper airway structures in obstructive sleep apnea. Sleep 2010;33(9):1249–54.

51. Cistulli PA, Palmisano RG, Poole MD. Treatment of obstructive sleep apnea syndrome by rapid maxillary expansion. Sleep 1998;21(8):831–5.

52. Singh GD, Griffin TM, Chandrashekhar R. Biomimetic oral appliance therapy in adults with mild to moderate obstructive sleep apnea. Austin J Sleep Disord 2014;1(1):1–5. Available at: http://austinpublishinggroup.org/sleep-disorders/. Accessed April 18, 2016.

53. El-Solh AA, Moitheennazima B, Akinnusi ME, et al. Combined oral appliance and positive airway pressure therapy for obstructive sleep apnea: a pilot study. Sleep Breath 2011;15(2):203–8.

Novel Surgical Approaches for the Treatment of Obstructive Sleep Apnea

Ryan J. Soose, MD

KEYWORDS

- Sleep apnea • Sleep surgery • Palate surgery • Expansion pharyngoplasty
- Upper airway stimulation • Hypoglossal nerve stimulation • Drug-induced sleep endoscopy

KEY POINTS

- Drug-induced sedation endoscopy provides diagnostic information about the anatomic structures, locations, and patterns of collapse under conditions that more closely resemble sleep rather than wakefulness.
- Improved phenotyping of the muscular and skeletal anatomy allows for integration of this anatomy into a customized medical and/or surgical treatment plan.
- Advanced palatal surgery techniques are now available that use more reconstructive and physiologically sound (rather than excisional) techniques to improve effectiveness and reduce morbidity.
- Upper airway neurostimulation therapy via an implantable hypoglossal nerve stimulation system has been shown to provide sustainable multilevel treatment of selected patients with moderate to severe obstructive sleep apnea with low morbidity and good adherence.

INTRODUCTION: THE ROLE OF SURGICAL THERAPY

Surgical therapy for obstructive sleep apnea (OSA) has traditionally been synonymous with uvulopalatopharyngoplasty (UPPP) from the perspective of many practicing sleep specialists as well as their patients. However, sleep-disordered breathing surgery encompasses dozens of surgical procedures and approaches for a wide variety of clinical applications:

- First-line surgical therapy to address intraluminal obstructing lesions, such as adenotonsillectomy in pediatric OSA
- Minimally invasive outpatient procedures for nonapneic snoring or upper airway resistance syndrome
- Nasal surgery to lower nasal airway resistance and augment the effectiveness of positive pressure or oral appliance therapy
- Hypoglossal nerve stimulation (HNS) therapy to augment the neuromuscular activity of the pharynx
- Multilevel upper airway reconstructive pharyngeal surgery as salvage after failure of medical device treatments
- Skeletal advancement surgery for patients with maxillomandibular deficiency or as salvage treatment
- Bariatric surgery to facilitate substantial weight loss
- Tracheotomy to bypass upper airway obstruction

Disclosure Statement: Consultant for Inspire Medical Systems and Investigator in the Inspire STAR Trial.
UPMC Division of Sleep Surgery, Department of Otolaryngology, University of Pittsburgh School of Medicine, UPMC Mercy Building B, Suite 11500, 1400 Locust Street, Pittsburgh, PA 15219, USA
E-mail address: sooserj@upmc.edu

Sleep Med Clin 11 (2016) 189–202
http://dx.doi.org/10.1016/j.jsmc.2016.01.006

For the millions of patients who will not accept or are unable to adhere to positive pressure therapy (continuous positive airway pressure [CPAP]), surgical therapy can provide a method of symptom and quality-of-life improvement in addition to a reduction in cardiovascular risk. Surgical treatment of OSA has evolved rapidly over the last decade. Improved understanding of the pathophysiology of OSA and improved methods of airway evaluation, endoscopically and radiographically, have resulted in better phenotyping the various anatomic patterns of collapse and subsequent customization of novel surgical approaches.

Numerous modifications and advances in pharyngeal and skeletal surgical techniques have been reported around the world in the last decade. In addition, new implantable device technologies that use novel approaches to stabilize the airway continue to be developed every year. A comprehensive review of all such procedures and devices is beyond the scope of this article. The goal of this article, rather, is to highlight a few select novel diagnostic and therapeutic surgical approaches.

Novel Diagnostic Evaluation Approach

Drug-induced sedation endoscopy

Background By definition, almost all patients with OSA have some form of anatomic vulnerability of the upper airway. Successful OSA surgical therapy depends critically on proper knowledge and phenotyping of the upper airway structure and subsequently integrating that anatomy into surgical decision-making. Physical examination, lateral cephalometric radiograph, computed tomography scan, MRI, awake flexible nasolaryngoscopy, acoustic analysis, manometry, and drug-induced sedation endoscopy (DISE) represent some of the options available to better phenotype the structural anatomy of the upper airway.[1] One of the major limitations of most airway assessment techniques is that the information is usually obtained while patients are awake and upright, not in a sleep-disordered breathing state.

DISE allows for dynamic examination of the airway during conditions that more closely resemble the reduced upper airway dilator muscle activity and loss of control of breathing that occurs during sleep.[2] When performed under specific conditions and guidelines, propofol-induced sedation correlates most closely with deeper levels (stage N2) of non–rapid eye movement (NREM) sleep and maintains a similar AHI as compared with physiologic sleep.[3,4] Studies of sleep endoscopy have demonstrated validity, test-retest

reliability, and interrater reliability.[5,6] Recent data suggest that utilization of DISE can improve treatment outcomes with oral appliances.[7–9] Evidence is emerging that certain DISE findings are related to treatment outcome and that DISE is a valuable selection tool in treatment decision-making.[10–15] Approximately 100 articles have been published on DISE just in the last 5 years. The recently published European position paper provides a comprehensive review and starting point for the reader interested in more in-depth analysis of the data and controversies surrounding DISE.[16]

Technique The goal of sedated endoscopy is to examine and phenotype the upper airway structure under conditions that more closely resemble sleep rather than wakefulness. Although the procedure was first described by Croft and Pringle in 199,[17] the foundation for the current procedure was established by Hillman and others[2] a decade or two later. Using the bispectral index score (BIS) monitor and a slow gradual propofol infusion (no benzodiazepine, no bolus), they demonstrated a nonlinear increase in upper airway collapsibility (pharyngeal critical pressure [Pcrit]) and decrease in genioglossus muscle activity occurring in a relatively narrow BIS range.[2]

The procedure is commonly performed in an outpatient surgery setting or bronchoscopy suite with standard anesthesia monitoring, including oxygen saturation, electrocardiogram, and blood pressure. In the author's medical center, patients receive an intravenous catheter in the preoperative area and glycopyrrolate to reduce secretions. Once in the surgical suite, patients remain on the same mobile bed where a BIS monitor and the standard anesthesia monitors are placed. One side of the nose is anesthetized and decongested with topical lidocaine and oxymetazoline. A slow gradual propofol infusion is initiated with a standardized protocol to titrate to clinical signs of sedation and sleep-disordered breathing as well as to a BIS level between 50 and 70.

The flexible endoscope is then inserted to examine both sides of the nose and the pharynx and larynx under the conditions that mimic sleep. When the steady state of snoring and obstructive sleep-disordered breathing is achieved (usually 5–10 minutes), the anatomic locations and pattern of collapse are recorded at baseline and again during other iterations as dictated by patients' clinical history (eg, with jaw advancement, with patients' own mandibular repositioning device in place, with changes in neck position). In patients with persistent AHI elevation on CPAP or other symptoms concerning for inadequate effectiveness of CPAP despite regular use, DISE can also be performed with patients' CPAP on. The flexible endoscope may be inserted in through the CPAP mask interface via a bronchoscopy elbow connector.

Phenotyping the upper airway The findings may be scored with one of the available staging systems, such as the velum oropharynx tongue-base epiglottis or the nose oropharynx hypopharynx and larynx classification.[18,19] The goal of the endoscopic examination is to phenotype the pharyngeal muscle buttress system (**Fig. 1**), which may have a different length, anterior-posterior (AP) depth, lateral dimension, and structural elements in each patient. The anatomy of this pharyngeal muscle buttress system consists of the palatopharyngeus and levator palatinus muscles as well as the tensor palatini, palatoglossus, salpingopharyngeus, and uvular muscles and is further influenced and determined by the craniofacial structure within which it sits as well as the degree of jaw laxity, neck position, and body position. A comprehensive staging system to capture and categorize all of the various anatomic phenotypes does not yet exist; however, the current knowledge and staging systems at least provide a framework to more accurately describe the anatomic patterns of collapse above and beyond the historical and inadequate site or level of obstruction.

One example of the different palatal phenotypes that can be described with DISE is shown in **Fig. 2**. Although significant heterogeneity exists regarding the palatal anatomy, the pattern of palatal obstruction is often described in reference to 2 ends of a spectrum: AP collapse versus complete concentric collapse (CCC). The classic end of the AP spectrum is a palate with maxillary retrusion and subsequent in the AP dimension at the level of the maxilla, the levator palatine muscle sling (genu), and the velum, often with a long vertical segment of soft palate. In its classic form, the CCC end of the spectrum, on the other hand, involves a wide open maxilla and open genu, with a more oblique or horizontally oriented soft palate that obstructs distally at the velum because of large lateral oropharyngeal walls. Similar descriptions of tongue base phenotypes and other anatomic variations of the upper airway during DISE have also been described.[20-22]

Using DISE or other phenotyping modalities to differentiate seems to have treatment implications. For example, for the palate description earlier, CCC has been correlated with poorer outcomes with HNS therapy and remains an exclusion criterion for the current Food and Drug Administration (FDA)–approved implantable neurostimulation system.[23] Furthermore, when considering reconstructive surgical options, maxillary advancement or transpalatal advancement surgery would be more conducive to addressing the classic AP pattern of retropalatal collapse with maxillary retrusion, whereas expansion sphincter pharyngoplasty (ESP) (discussed later) or other lateral pharyngoplasty techniques have been shown to more successfully address the CCC anatomy.

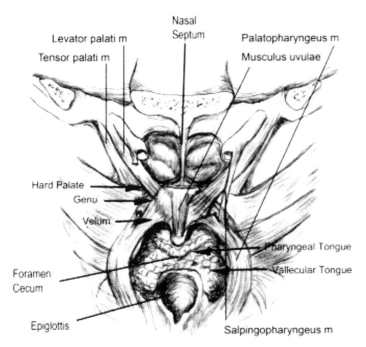

Fig. 1. The pharyngeal muscle buttress system. The posterior view of the pharynx depicts selected major muscle groups (anatomic landmarks) that define the lumen. The nasal septum allows identification of the posterior hard palate and the superior border of the soft palate. The levator palatini muscle describes the central soft palate, whereas the velum defines the inferior soft palate. The lateral walls of the velopharynx may be defined by the palatopharyngeus muscles (or superior pole of the palatine tonsils, if present). The lower pharynx anterior wall border is described by the pharyngeal tongue, vallecular tongue, and epiglottis. m, muscle. (*From* Woodson BT. A method to describe the pharyngeal airway. Laryngoscope 2015;125(5):1234; with permission.)

Levator palati m
Tensor palati m
Nasal Septum
Palatopharyngeus m
Musculus uvulae
Hard Palate
Genu
Velum
Pharyngeal Tongue
Vallecular Tongue
Foramen Cecum
Epiglottis
Salpingopharyngeus m

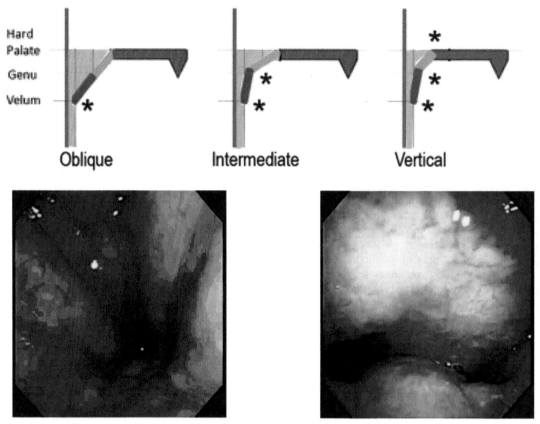

Fig. 2. Anatomic patterns of palatal collapse during DISE. Narrowing (*asterisks*) occurs in the upper pharynx at the following locations: oblique pattern at the velum; intermediate at the velum and genu; and the vertical at velum, genu, and hard palate. Complete concentric collapse of the obliquely oriented soft palate is shown in the endoscopic image on the left, and the AP pattern of a more vertically oriented soft palate is shown in the endoscopic image on the right. (*From* Woodson BT. A method to describe the pharyngeal airway. Laryngoscope 2015;125(5):1235; with permission.)

Indications Debate still exists on the precise indications for DISE. DISE may be performed in any clinical situation whereby a more thorough evaluation of the upper airway structure and patterns of collapse are needed for investigation into the structural components of patients' OSA pathophysiology and for patient counseling and treatment planning. Examples of commonly used clinical applications are as follows:

- To plan a multilevel upper airway surgical plan in patients who have failed medical device therapy and present with concern for multilevel or multifactorial airway collapsibility
- To evaluate the upper airway after prior failure of airway reconstructive surgery
- To evaluate for anatomic candidacy for HNS therapy
- At the time of staged or adjunctive nasal surgery, DISE to evaluate the rest of the upper airway anatomy should additional surgical considerations be needed in the future

- In patients who achieve partial but incomplete results with oral appliance therapy, DISE with and without the oral appliance to evaluate for residual locations of collapse, and additional medical or surgical treatment options to further augment the effectiveness of the oral appliance
- In patients with persistent AHI elevation or other evidence of airway obstruction despite CPAP use; DISE with and without the CPAP in place to investigate the reasons for CPAP failure, such as epiglottic collapse or iatrogenic airway obstruction due to the interface impact on the jaw and neck position

Future Although DISE is currently the most widely used diagnostic tool for upper airway endoscopic evaluation of patients with OSA, consensus is still lacking on the exact protocol used for sedation, the clinical indications for when it should be performed, the staging system to report findings, and how to translate the DISE findings into proper procedure selection. Future research is needed to standardize the DISE sedation and procedure protocol, to better define the staging of the upper airway anatomy, to quantify findings, and to determine the role of DISE in the evaluation and titration of adjustable therapies, such as oral appliance therapy and positional therapy and HNS therapy. Perhaps the most important goal of future research is to determine whether DISE actually favorably improves OSA outcomes.

Novel Airway Surgery Approach

Expansion sphincter pharyngoplasty

Background Most physicians are familiar with the general concept of UPPP. Palatal obstruction has been documented to be at least a contributing factor in most patients with OSA; therefore, palatal surgery plays a role in surgical therapy, particularly in those patients who fail other forms of medical therapy. Fujita and colleagues[24] first described traditional UPPP in 1981, the same year that CPAP was introduced. Although not as much was known at the time about the pathophysiology or cardiovascular sequelae of OSA, it represented a major treatment advance because, before 1981, tonsillectomy and tracheotomy were essentially the only known effective surgical therapies. In its classic form, this ablative procedure essentially involves en-bloc resection of the tonsils, uvula, and random portions of the soft palate mucosa, glandular tissue, and muscles.

Until recently, this particular procedure was largely unchanged and surgical series resulted in mediocre results at best, particularly when used as a sole procedure. In 1996, Sher and colleagues[25] attempted to summarize UPPP efficacy with a review of 37 articles and approximately 500 patients who underwent surgical therapy for OSA. These surgical series were hampered by poorly defined inclusion/selection criteria, variable surgical technique, and inconsistent follow-up. Surgical success was defined as a postoperative respiratory disturbance index less than 20 with at least a 50% reduction from baseline or an apnea index less than 10 with at least a 50% reduction from baseline. Summarizing the data from these 500+ patients, a 41% success rate was reported.[25] Although similar to long-term acceptable compliance rates with other forms of medical therapy, the overall results were suboptimal.

Need for procedure modifications

Improving effectiveness Multiple prior studies of cases of UPPP failure have arrived at strikingly similar conclusions. Whether using imaging, manometry, or video endoscopic techniques, approximately 84% of patients who have persistent disease after traditional UPPP have been shown to still have significant obstruction at the retropalatal portion of the airway.[26] In 1998, Langin aimed to evaluate the impact of UPPP on upper airway anatomy by posing the following questions: (1) Does traditional UPPP actually enlarge the oropharyngeal airway? (2) Could the outcome of UPPP be explained in terms of the morphologic modifications produced by the surgery? Those patients who responded to palatal surgery with a successful reduction in the AHI (13 → 4) had a significant increase in the cross-sectional area at the level of the oropharynx. In contrast, the nonresponders (AHI 14 → 25) had no change in the cross-sectional area, or in some cases even a smaller retropalatal airway, after palatal surgery.[27]

These findings reinforce the idea that it is not simply the level of obstruction that predicts surgical success; rather, it is the specific pattern of obstruction, proper selection of the specific type of palatal surgery, and proper execution of the surgical technique that determine results. In other words, just because patients with palatal airway obstruction undergo a palatal procedure does not mean that the palatal airway was adequately enlarged or stabilized.

Reducing morbidity Effectiveness is not the only factor driving the decision for surgery. Perioperative morbidity, side effects, and risk are just as important. Tracheotomy and bimaxillary advancement are quite effective, but the associated morbidity precludes use in most patients. Serious perioperative complications of palatal surgery are uncommon (~1%) even in a large US Department of Veterans Affairs patient population with a high incidence of smoking.[28] Nevertheless, other side effects, such as globus sensation, mucous feeling, dry throat, and change in voice/swallowing, may be relatively common and underreported with traditional UPPP. These side effects can be quite bothersome to patients and potentially irreversible.

These benign, but often underreported, side effects may be significantly lessened by newer techniques and instrumentation designed to preserve mucosa, limit collateral thermal damage, and improve postoperative medical therapy. One of the most important changes, however, that may dramatically reduce morbidity and improve postoperative recovery and function is the preservation of the uvula. Although traditional UPPP techniques involve resection of the entire structure of the uvula, current understanding of pharyngeal physiology suggests that the uvula is an important physiologic structure rather than part of the airway problem in sleep apnea.

The uvular submucosa has a uniquely extensive immune cell population (primarily mast cells) that is important for the immunologic induction of mucosal tolerance to inhaled and ingested antigens.[29] The uvula has one of the highest concentrations of type II, fast-twitch muscle fibers in the human body, which are essential for the quick coordinated movements of speech and swallowing function. Its glandular area also comprises the highest concentration of serous glands (as opposed to mucous glands) in the oral cavity and oropharynx. The storage ducts are capable of quickly secreting, via muscle contraction, large volumes of serous fluid.[30] With video endoscopic techniques, Back and colleagues[31] demonstrated that the uvula plays an essential role in basting the posterior pharyngeal wall with thin serous saliva. These findings likely explain the local pharyngeal side effects that occur in many patients undergoing traditional UPPP and in part serve as the basis for the development of newer, less morbid, and more effective palatal surgical procedures.

Indications As discussed in the DISE section, proper procedure selection and execution integrally depend on knowledge of the anatomy and physiology of the upper airway. The expansion pharyngoplasty is ideally suited to patients with a more obliquely or horizontally oriented soft palate, with no significant maxillary skeletal deficiency, and with large lateral oropharyngeal walls resulting in concentric pattern of obstruction at the distal soft palate.

Surgical technique The surgical technique was originally described in 2007 by Pang and Woodson[32] and represented ongoing modifications of the lateral pharyngoplasty techniques previously described (**Fig. 3**). If present, the tonsils are first removed with maximal mucosal preservation. The palatopharyngeus muscles, which primarily account for the enlarged and medialized lateral pharyngeal walls, are dissected free from the posterior tonsillar pillars and rotated as bilateral pedicled muscle flaps toward the hamulus. The effect is an anterior, superior, and lateral vector of pull on the velum resulting in enlargement and stabilization of the lateral dimension of the retropalatal space (**Fig. 4**). Additional contouring of the uvula and velum can be combined with the expansion pharyngoplasty; however, the bulk of the uvular structure and function is preserved. As opposed to the *excisional*, or even destructive, approach of the traditional UPPP, the ESP uses a *reconstructive* approach with a muscle flap suspension technique.

Outcomes data A prospective randomized study in 2007 compared the effectiveness of ESP with the traditional UPPP.[32] Forty-five patients with moderate to severe OSA, CPAP intolerance, small tonsils, Friedman tongue position II or III, body mass index (BMI) less than 30 kg/m², and lateral oropharyngeal wall collapse were randomized to either ESP or UPPP. Surgical success was defined by polysomnographic evidence of AHI reduction to the mild or normal range and at least a 50% reduction. Success rates were significantly higher in the ESP group (78%), compared with the traditional UPPP group (45%), which more closely resembled Sher and colleagues[25] published historical success rates. A more recent meta-analysis of 5 ESP studies reported a mean AHI reduction from 40.0 ±12.6 at baseline to 8.3 ±5.2 postoperatively. The overall prorated pooled success rate for all the patients was 86.3% and was substantially higher than the success rates reported for control groups or historical data on traditional UPPP techniques.[33]

Future Although on an anecdotal level, postoperative morbidity is also better with ESP compared with UPPP, further studies are needed to demonstrate whether the advanced palatal surgery modifications result in reduced pain, swallowing dysfunction, dryness, or other pharyngeal side effects. Future investigation is also needed to determine the most appropriate patient and phenotype selection, to better standardize surgical technique, and to examine the role of ESP in combination with other medical and/or surgical treatments, such as oral appliance therapy and HNS therapy.

Novel Therapeutic Approach

Hypoglossal nerve stimulation therapy
Background There is increasing evidence that the neuromuscular control of breathing during sleep plays a key role in the sleep-disordered breathing pathophysiology for many patients with OSA.[34] Traditional upper airway surgery procedures, and even much of the medical device therapy available, primarily target the anatomic vulnerability. A simplified version of the upper airway neuromuscular feedback loop has been described with afferents from the pharynx, through the superior laryngeal nerve, to the nucleus solitaries and efferents from the hypoglossal nerve motor nucleus to the genioglossus muscle.[35] The genioglossus muscle is the primary upper airway dilator muscle and in normal healthy subjects responds to negative intraluminal pressure with a corresponding increase in genioglossus electromyographic (EMG) activity. This negative pressure reflex seems to be dysfunctional in many patients with OSA.

Interestingly, patients with OSA actually exhibit elevated genioglossus muscle EMG activity

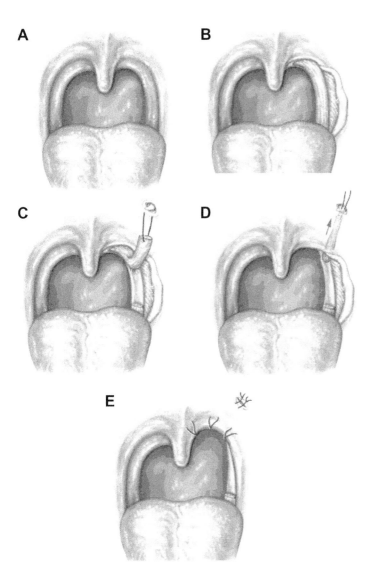

Fig. 3. ESP technique. The tonsils are removed with maximal mucosal preservation (A) followed by identification and dissection of the palatopharyngeus muscle in the posterior tonsillar pillar (B). The palatopharyngeus muscle is then elevated as a pedicled muscle flap toward its insertion into the soft palate (C). The flap is pulled through a submucosal tunnel and out through a separate stab incision adjacent to the hamulus where it is anchored to the fibrous tissue of the lateral soft palate (D). The resultant effect is an anterior, superior, and lateral vector of pull on the soft palate to enlarge the lateral dimension of the retropalatal space (E). (From Woodson BT, Sitton M, jacobowitz O. Expansion sphincter pharyngoplasty and palatal advancement pharyngoplasty: airway evaluation and surgical techniques. Operative Tech Otolaryngol 2012;23:6; with permission.)

during wakefulness compared with healthy controls.[36] This phenomenon in patients with OSA has long been attributed to compensation for a narrower and more collapsible airway. Recent data suggest that it is a manifestation of neuromuscular dysfunction with EMG patterns similar to denervation/renervation injury.[37] The cause of the neuromuscular dysfunction is unclear but may be related to intermittent hypoxia, systemic inflammation, or possibly vibrational trauma from snoring. A hypoglossal nerve conduction study in 16 patients with OSA reported delayed distal latency in 75% and low motor amplitude in 100%, compared with normative data, suggesting that neuromuscular dysfunction of the upper airway may be part of the pathophysiology and/or a consequence of untreated OSA.[38] Augmenting the efferent limb of the neuromuscular

feedback loop by stimulating the hypoglossal nerve, or the genioglossus muscle directly, may provide a therapeutic mechanism for some patients with OSA.

Electrical stimulation of the upper airway Decades of animal studies demonstrated that electrical stimulation of the hypoglossal nerve was feasible and produced corresponding increases in airflow and airway stability.[39–41] Although initial studies bore mixed results regarding the tolerability of electrical stimulation, multiple human studies confirmed that HNS improves airflow and upper airway stability, without causing arousal from sleep or adverse neuromuscular side effects, and can provide a treatment of OSA.[42–44] Oliven and colleagues[45] demonstrated the airway effects of selective stimulation of protrusor and retrusor muscles. Selective

A

Preoperative   Postoperative

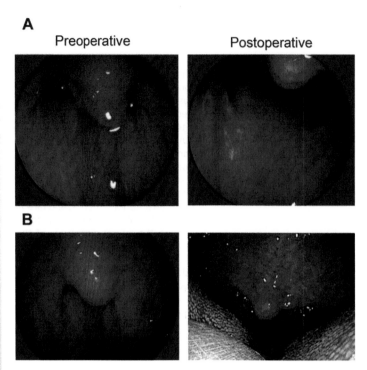

B

Fig. 4. Anatomic effect of the ESP: preoperative versus postoperative. (*A*) A 70° telescope view from the oropharynx into the retropalatal space. Note the enlargement in the lateral and AP dimensions of the velopharynx and tenting of the pharyngeal mucosa laterally. (*B*) A 0° telescope view from the oral cavity before and 3 months after ESP. ESP is associated with increased lateral oropharyngeal dimension while still preserving the uvula and soft palate mucosa and muscle.

intramuscular stimulation of the genioglossus significantly lowered Pcrit (more stable airway), whereas selective stimulation of the styloglossus and hyoglossus increased Pcrit (more collapsible airway). Coactivation of both protrusor and retrusor muscles resulted in a net improvement in airflow and reduction in Pcrit confirming that the genioglossus is the dominant upper airway muscle. Nasopharyngoscopy was used to demonstrate that genioglossus stimulation can result in enlargement and stabilization of not only the retrolingual portion of the airway but also the retropalatal space (see **Fig. 1**). As OSA frequently involves multilevel collapsibility, this was a key observation suggesting that HNS has the potential to impact multiple levels of the pharyngeal airway rather than the tongue base alone.

Human pilot and feasibility studies The wealth of animal and human basic science data was then combined with existing implantable neurostimulation technology from other medical applications to develop the first implantable HNS for OSA. A pilot study published in 2001 reported on 8 participants receiving an implantable HNS system consisting of a tripolar cuff electrode, an implantable pulse generator, and a chest wall respiratory pressure sensor (**Fig. 5**).[46] There were no reported serious adverse events, and stimulation did not cause arousals from sleep or negatively alter tongue function. The mean AHI reduced significantly; but

despite the encouraging results, electrode breakage and sensor malfunction occurred in several participants, precluding use beyond the 6-month study period.

Following the published technical limitations of the human pilot study, multiple investigators and medical device companies spent a decade improving the product before the launch of 2 larger trials with results available as of 2011.[47,48] One of the feasibility studies reported AHI less than 50, BMI 32 kg/m^2 or less, and absence of complete concentric pattern of collapse at the palate were predictors of therapy response. Eight additional participants were then enrolled prospectively with the aforementioned clinical inclusion criteria and demonstrated significant AHI reduction from 38.9 ±9.8 to 10.0 ±11.0 (*P*<.01) at the 6-month postimplant visit. In 2013, Vanderveken and colleagues[23] also studied the predictive value of DISE in assessing therapeutic response to implanted upper airway stimulation (UAS) for participants with OSA. The researchers concluded that the absence of palatal complete circumferential collapse during DISE may predict therapeutic success with implanted UAS therapy.

Anatomic effect on the upper airway The potential success of the HNS therapy seemed to hinge on 2 key factors: (1) The first factor is the ability of the therapy to provide *multilevel* upper airway improvement. Imaging, fluoroscopy, and DISE

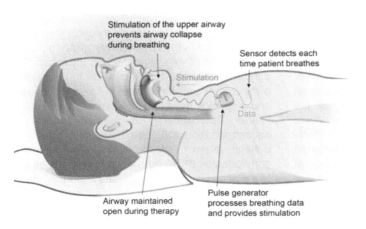

Stimulation of the upper airway prevents airway collapse during breathing

Sensor detects each time patient breathes

Stimulation

Data

Airway maintained open during therapy

Pulse generator processes breathing data and provides stimulation

Fig. 5. Implantable upper airway stimulation system. The HNS system consists of 3 implanted components: (1) an implantable pulse generator in a subcutaneous pocket in the right upper chest, (2) a stimulation lead with a cuff electrode placed on the medial branch of the hypoglossal nerve in the right submandibular space, and (3) a sensing lead to detect ventilatory effort placed in the intercostal space facing the pleura. (*Courtesy of* Inspire Medical Systems, Minneapolis (MN), with permission.)

evaluation demonstrated that therapy responders, HNS therapy resulted in enlargement of the retropalatal space as well as the retrolingual portion of the airway (**Fig. 6**). Anterior displacement of the hyoid bone also occurred in most participants. This multilevel improvement may be due to several factors but is primarily thought to occur from the mechanical coupling of the tongue and palate via the palatoglossal and palatopharyngeus muscles. (2) The second factor is the ability to adjust and titrate the therapy. Unlike traditional sleep apnea surgery, HNS therapy can be titrated in the clinical or sleep laboratory setting to optimize effectiveness and comfort and graded response to increasing amplitude. Prior studies have shown a graded increase in airflow and airway measurements with increasing stimulation amplitudes.[49,50]

Surgical technique For the current FDA-approved device, the implantation consists of an approximately 2-hour outpatient procedure under general anesthesia. Fine-wire electrodes are placed in the genioglossus muscle and the hyoglossus/styloglossus muscles for intraoperative nerve monitoring. After standard sterile prep and drape, a small incision is made in the right upper neck parallel to a natural skin crease and carried down to the floor of the submandibular triangle where the hypoglossal nerve is identified. Nerve monitoring is used to selectively capture the distal tongue protrusor branches supplying the genioglossus muscle activity and to exclude branches innervating the tongue retractor muscles. The stimulation cuff electrode is placed around the distal protrusor branches and secured to the digastric tendon.

Stimulation OFF   Stimulation ON

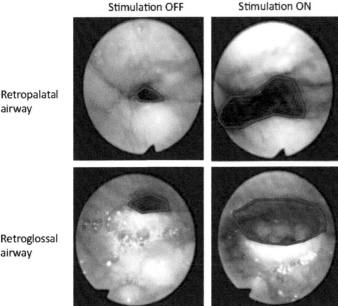

Retropalatal airway

Retroglossal airway

Fig. 6. The multilevel effect of UAS during DISE. The outlined areas demonstrate the increase in cross-sectional area of both the retropalatal and retrolingual portions of the upper airway with HNS therapy. (*From* Dedhia RC, Strollo PJ, Soose RJ. Upper airway stimulation therapy: past, present, and future. Sleep 2015;38:900; with permission.)

A second incision is made in the right lateral chest wall for placement of the pleural respiratory sensor. The sensor is inserted, facing the pleura, into a tunnel between the external and internal intercostal muscles in approximately the fifth or sixth intercostal space and secured to the chest wall. The sensing lead and stimulation lead are each then tunneled into a subcutaneous pocket in right upper chest and connected to the implantable pulse generator (IPG), which is secured to the pectoralis fascia. After good confirmation of tongue protrusion visually and electrically, as well as good sensing waveform, the wounds are closed and the procedure is completed. Unlike anatomy-altering traditional sleep surgery procedures, most patients can be safely discharged home the same day given the lack of airway surgery, the minimal/no opioid pain medication use, and absence of significant obesity per the screening criteria.

Follow-up Patients return to the outpatient sleep clinic approximately 1 month postoperatively for device activation. At this time, electrical thresholds are established and programmed. Patients are provided the remote control and educated on how to use the therapy. At bedtime, the remote is placed over the IPG in the right upper chest to turn the device on. After a predetermined delay time to allow for sleep onset (eg, 30 minutes), the therapy syncs with the respiratory cycle and rhythmically activates the upper airway dilator muscles from the end of expiration through the inspiratory period. The remote allows patients to have complete control over the therapy with on, off, pause, and amplitude adjustment available.

After approximately a 1-month period of accommodation and self-titration of the therapy, patients return to the sleep laboratory for polysomnography (PSG) both to (1) assess the objective outcomes of the therapy and (2) further titrate therapy for optimal comfort and effectiveness (**Fig. 7**). Patients are then transitioned to long-term follow-up in the sleep medicine clinic to monitor adherence, side effects, and subjective outcomes, similar to longitudinal management of CPAP. The physician programmer is used in the clinic setting to sync with the device, monitor objective adherence data, and to make stimulation parameter adjustments as needed. The current IPG battery life is expected to last at least 10 years, at which point the battery may be changed.

Indications All patients being considered for HNS therapy must undergo a standard comprehensive sleep medicine evaluation and upper airway surgical consultation. According to the

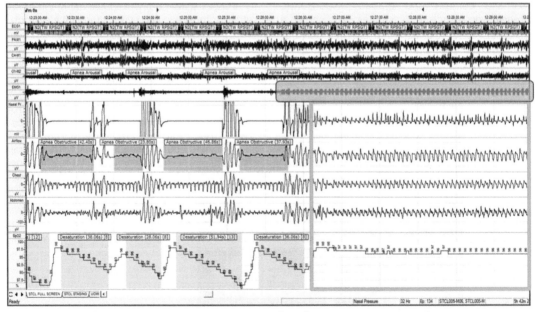

Fig. 7. Titration of UAS therapy during PSG. PSG snapshot showing an approximately 6-minute respiratory window. The left side of the image shows periodic airflow limitation, fluctuating respiratory effort, and associated oxygen desaturations consistent with OSA. Device activation is illustrated by the green box. After the device synchronizes with ventilatory effort, immediate improvement in control of breathing and oximetry is observed. (*From* Dedhia RC, Strollo PJ, Soose RJ. Upper airway stimulation therapy: past, present, and future. Sleep 2015;38:904; with permission.)

current FDA-approved guidelines, HNS therapy is indicated for patients with the following:

- Moderate to severe OSA
- Intolerance or inadequate adherence with CPAP
- BMI ≤32
- Absence of complete concentric pattern of retropalatal collapse on DISE

These inclusion criteria represent an oversimplification of the screening process and must be taken into the clinical context of the rest of patients' sleep medicine history, comorbid sleep or medical disorders, craniofacial and upper airway anatomy, and other confounding factors. More data from other clinical trials and the increasing clinical experience worldwide are needed to produce further refinements in indications and patient selection.

Data from the stimulation therapy for apnea reduction trial The basic science experiments and feasibility studies served as the basis for the multicenter prospective Stimulation Therapy for Apnea Reduction (STAR) trial.[51] Eligible implant participants had moderate to severe OSA, CPAP intolerance, BMI of 32 or less, and absence of a complete circumferential pattern of palatal obstruction on DISE. After a rigorous clinical, polysomnographic, and DISE screening, 126 participants underwent surgical implantation of the HNS system and were followed for at least 12 months to assess effectiveness and adverse events. Devices were titrated in the sleep laboratory during full-montage attended polysomnography, similar to CPAP titration, to optimize comfort and effectiveness. Primary outcome measures (AHI, 4% oxygen desaturation index [ODI]) and secondary outcomes measures (Epworth Sleepiness Scale [ESS], Functional Outcomes of Sleep Questionnaire [FOSQ]) all demonstrated clinically and statistically significant improvements at 12 months (median AHI reduction from 29.3 to 9.0 and median ODI reduction from 25.4 to 7.4). Two-thirds of the implanted participants were considered successful responders to therapy by previously published surgical success criteria (median AHI 30 → 6). Quality-of-life measures also improved significantly across the cohort with ESS reduced from median 11.0 to 6.0 and FOSQ increased from 14.6 to 18.2 at the 12-month follow-up.

Risk and morbidity data were favorable with no permanent hypoglossal nerve weakness, no serious device-related infection requiring explantation, and significantly less postoperative discomfort compared with traditional pharyngeal or skeletal sleep apnea surgeries. One-third of the participants reported intermittent and self-limited tongue discomfort due to stimulation itself or abrasion of the tongue on an adjacent tooth. Adherence was excellent by self-report (86% of participants using the therapy nightly at the 12-month mark), but detailed objective data monitoring were limited.

At 12 months, a randomized therapy withdrawal study was performed in the first 46 responders, similar to prior withdrawal studies that have been performed using nasal CPAP.[52] As with CPAP withdrawal studies, this study demonstrated that withdrawal of HNS therapy resulted in a recurrence of OSA severity, daytime sleepiness, and impaired quality of life. These results emphasize that, similar to CPAP, nightly use of the therapy is required to maintain effectiveness. Additional studies on long-term outcomes have since been published from the STAR trial. At 18 months' follow-up, PSG outcome measures were maintained without an increase of the stimulation thresholds or tongue injury.[53]

At 24 months' follow-up, UAS was reported to provide clinically meaningful and statistically significant improvements in patient-centered OSA outcome measures, including snoring, daytime sleepiness, and sleep-related quality of life.[54] The effect size on patient-centered outcome measures was also large and compared favorably with CPAP as well as other second-line therapies. Finally, the significant improvements in both subjective and objective outcome measures were maintained at 3 years' follow-up. A total of 116 participants (92%) completed the scheduled 36-month clinical follow-up, and 98 participants (78%) completed a voluntary 36-month PSG. For the group undergoing the 36-month PSG, 74% met responder status.[55]

Discussion
Comparison of upper airway stimulation to other obstructive sleep apnea treatments UAS is titratable and adjustable, similar to CPAP or even oral appliances, with multiple device parameters that can be modified postoperatively. A variety of configurations (eg, bipolar vs monopolar, pulse width, amplitude, duration of stimulation, timing with respiration) may be programmed to optimize therapy effectiveness as well as patient comfort/adherence. Similar to a positive pressure titration study, the UAS device is titrated at real-time during overnight PSG using a wireless telemetry unit. This adjustability of the therapy, in conjunction with the expected 10+ year battery life, may be particularly important because OSA is most commonly a chronic long-term condition that requires continued reevaluation and management throughout the life span. Device interrogation in

the office provides adherence monitoring akin to CPAP data download technology. UAS therapy puts the sleep medicine physician and the sleep laboratory technician at the center of this longitudinal care model.

UAS also differs from traditional OSA airway surgery in several positive ways. It provides multilevel airway improvement with only one procedure as evidenced by DISE studies demonstrating enlargement of the retropalatal space as well as the retrolingual space. The implant does not alter upper airway anatomy and is technically reversible. Furthermore, unlike other tongue base or pharyngeal surgeries, UAS surgical procedure is completely external to the pharynx, thus, substantially reducing postoperative discomfort and recovery time and minimizing or even eliminating the traditional risks of throat hemorrhage, dysphagia, change in taste, or other untoward pharyngeal side effects of anatomy-altering procedures.

Future directions Based on the available data, particularly the results of the STAR trial, UAS therapy has a favorable risk-benefit profile and is well positioned as a second-line treatment of patients with moderate to severe OSA. Early cost-effectiveness analysis has been published; although upfront costs are higher, long-term cost-effectiveness data compare favorably with other OSA treatments, including CPAP.[56] More studies are needed to better understand which anatomic and pathophysiologic patient phenotypes will respond best to therapy. Further work is also needed to better define the most effective and appropriate stimulation parameters and titration protocols.

Other limitations include incompatibility of the current technology with MRI and the need for 3 external incisions for implantation, 2 factors that may preclude a subset of patients from considering this therapy. Continued efforts to produce a smaller MRI-compatible pulse generator, more advanced and user-friendly patient programmer, and more sophisticated and comprehensive data recording technology will further advance the treatment. Finally, the role of UAS in combination therapy needs to be explored, as a recent case report showed incremental benefit by combining UAS and a mandibular repositioning device.[57]

SUMMARY

The OSA treatment armamentarium is continuously evolving and expanding, both medically and surgically. Although CPAP remains the standard first-line therapy with the most robust data

on effectiveness, suboptimal adherence and acceptance rates necessitate consideration of alternative treatment strategies for many patients. Novel approaches to upper airway anatomic phenotyping, more reconstructive upper airway surgical techniques, and new implantable hypoglossal neurostimulation technology have very favorable potential to improve symptoms and quality-of-life measures, to reduce OSA disease severity and associated cardiovascular risk, and to serve as an adjunct to CPAP, oral appliances, and other forms of OSA medical therapy. Successful surgical therapy depends critically on accurate diagnosis, skillful knowledge and examination of the upper airway anatomy, proper procedure selection, and proficient technical application. The state-of-the-art approach centers on phenotyping each individual's multifactorial pattern of upper airway collapse and tailoring a multilevel, and often multimodality, treatment plan with effective, low morbidity, physiologically sound techniques rather than the sole site excisional model more commonly used over the past few decades.

REFERENCES

1. Stuck BA, Maurer JT. Airway evaluation in obstructive sleep apnea. Sleep Med Rev 2008;12(6):411–36.
2. Hillman DR, Walsh JH, Maddison KJ, et al. Evolution of changes in upper airway collapsibility during slow induction of anesthesia with propofol. Anesthesiology 2009;111:63–71.
3. Rabelo FA, Braga A, Kupper DS, et al. Propofol-induced sleep: polysomnographic evaluation of patients with obstructive sleep apnea and controls. Otolaryngol Head Neck Surg 2010;142:218–24.
4. Carrasco Llatas M, Agostini Porras G, Cuesta Gonzalez MT, et al. Drug-induced sleep endoscopy: a two drug comparison and simultaneous polysomnography. Eur Arch Otorhinolaryngol 2013;271:181–7.
5. Rodriguez-Bruno K, Goldberg AN, McCulloch CE, et al. Test-retest reliability of drug-induced sleep endoscopy. Otolaryngol Head Neck Surg 2009; 140:646–51.
6. Kezirian EJ, White DP, Malhotra A, et al. Interrater reliability of drug-induced sleep endoscopy. Arch Otolaryngol Head Neck Surg 2010;136(4): 393–7.
7. Johal A, Hector MP, Battagel JM, et al. Impact of sleep nasendoscopy on the outcome of mandibular advancement splint therapy in subjects with sleep-related breathing disorders. J Laryngol Otol 2007; 121:668–75.
8. Johal A, Battagel JM, Kotecha BT. Sleep nasendoscopy: a diagnostic tool for predicting treatment

success with mandibular advancement splints in obstructive sleep apnoea. Eur J Orthod 2005;27: 607–14.

9. Battagel JM, Johal A, Kotecha BT. Sleep nasendoscopy as a predictor of treatment success in snorers using mandibular advancement splints. J Laryngol Otol 2005;119:106–12.

10. Gillespie MB, Reddy RP, White DR, et al. A trial of drug-induced sleep endoscopy in the surgical management of sleep-disordered breathing. Laryngoscope 2013;123:277–82.

11. Eichler C, Sommer JU, Stuck BA, et al. Does drug-induced sleep endoscopy change the treatment concept of patients with snoring and obstructive sleep apnea? Sleep Breath 2013;17:63–8.

12. Iwanaga K, Hasegawa K, Shibata N, et al. Endoscopic examination of obstructive sleep apnea syndrome patients during drug-induced sleep. Acta Otolaryngol Suppl 2003;550:36–40.

13. Ravesloot MJL, de Vries N. One hundred consecutive patients undergoing drug-induced sleep endoscopy: results and evaluation. Laryngoscope 2011; 121:2710–6.

14. Koutsourelakis I, Safiruddin F, Ravesloot M, et al. Surgery for obstructive sleep apnea: sleep endoscopy determinants of outcome. Laryngoscope 2012;122:2587–91.

15. Kent DT, Rogers R, Soose RJ. Drug-induced sedation endoscopy in the evaluation of OSA patients with incomplete oral appliance therapy response. Otolaryngol Head Neck Surg 2015;153:302–7.

16. De Vito A, Carrasco Llatas M, Vanni A, et al. European position paper on drug-induced sedation endoscopy (DISE). Sleep Breath 2014;18:453–65.

17. Croft CB, Pringle M. Sleep nasendoscopy: a technique of assessment in snoring and obstructive sleep apnoea. Clin Otolaryngol Allied Sci 1991;16: 504–9.

18. Vicini C, De Vito A, Benazzo M, et al. The nose oropharynx hypopharynx and larynx (NOHL) classification: a new system of diagnostic standardized examination for OSAHS patients. Eur Arch Otorhinolaryngol 2012;269:1297–300.

19. Kezirian EJ, Hohenhorst W, de Vries N. Drug-induced sleep endoscopy: the VOTE classification. Eur Arch Otorhinolaryngol 2011;268:1233–6.

20. Woodson BT. A method to describe the pharyngeal airway. Laryngoscope 2015;125(5):1233–8.

21. Vroegop AV, Vanderveken OM, Boudewyns AN, et al. Drug-induced sleep endoscopy in sleep-disordered breathing: report on 1249 cases. Laryngoscope 2013;124:797–802.

22. Moore KE, Phillips C. A practical method for describing patterns of tongue-base narrowing (modification of Fujita) in awake adult patients with obstructive sleep apnea. J Oral Maxillofac Surg 2002;60:252–60.

23. Vanderveken OM, Maurer JT, Hohenhorst W, et al. Evaluation of drug-induced sleep endoscopy as a patient selection tool for implanted upper airway stimulation for obstructive sleep apnea. J Clin Sleep Med 2013;9:433–8.

24. Fujita S, Conway W, Zorick F, et al. Surgical correction of anatomic abnormalities in obstructive sleep apnea syndrome: uvulopalatopharyngoplasty. Otolaryngol Head Neck Surg 1981;89:923–34.

25. Sher AE, Schechtman KB, Piccirillo JF. The efficacy of surgical modifications of the upper airway in adults with obstructive sleep apnea. Sleep 1996; 19:156–77.

26. Woodson BT, Wooten MR. Manometric and endoscopic localization of airway obstruction after UPPP. Otolaryngol Head Neck Surg 1994; 111:38–43.

27. Langin T, Pepin J, Pendlebury S, et al. Upper airway changes in snorers and mild sleep apnea sufferers after UPPP. Chest 1998;113:1595–603.

28. Kezirian EJ, Weaver EM, Yueh B, et al. Incidence of serious complications after uvulopalatopharyngoplasty. Laryngoscope 2004;114:450–3.

29. Olofsson K, Mattsson C, Hammarstrom ML, et al. Human uvula: characterization of resident leukocytes and local cytokine production. Ann Otol Rhinol Laryngol 2000;109(5):488–96.

30. Finklestein Y, Meshorer A, Talmi YP, et al. The riddle of the uvula. Otolaryngol Head Neck Surg 1992;107: 444–51.

31. Back GW, Nadig S, Uppal S, et al. Why do we have a uvula?: literature review and a new theory. Clin Otolaryngol 2004;29:689–93.

32. Pang K, Woodson BT. Expansion sphincter pharyngoplasty: a new technique for the treatment of obstructive sleep apnea. Otolaryngol Head Neck Surg 2007;137:110–4.

33. Pang KP, Pang EB, Win MT, et al. Expansion sphincter pharyngoplasty for the treatment of OSA: a systematic review and meta-analysis. Eur Arch Otorhinolaryngol 2015. [Epub ahead of print].

34. Dempsey JA, Veasey SC, Morgan BJ, et al. Pathophysiology of sleep apnea. Physiol Rev 2010;90: 47–112.

35. White DP. Pathogenesis of obstructive and central sleep apnea. Am J Respir Crit Care Med 2005; 172:1363–70.

36. Mezzanotte WS, Tangel DJ, White DP. Waking genioglossal electromyogram in sleep apnea patients versus normal controls (a neuromuscular compensatory mechanism). J Clin Invest 1992;89:1571–9.

37. Saboisky JP, Butler JE, McKenzie DK, et al. Neural drive to human genioglossus in obstructive sleep apnoea. J Physiol 2007;585:135–46.

38. Ragab S. Hypoglossal nerve conduction studies in patients with obstructive sleep apnea. Egypt J Otolaryngol 2013;29:176–81.

39. Miki H, Hida W, Shindoh C, et al. Effects of electrical stimulation of the genioglossus on upper airway resistance in anesthetized dogs. Am Rev Respir Dis 1989;140:1279–84.

40. Yoo PB, Durand DM. Effects of selective hypoglossal nerve stimulation on canine upper airway mechanics. J Appl Physiol 2005;99:937–43.

41. Bishara H, Odeh M, Schnall RP, et al. Electrically-activated dilator muscles reduce pharyngeal resistance in anaesthetized dogs with upper airway obstruction. Eur Respir J 1995;8:1537–42.

42. Schwartz AR, Thut DC, Russ B, et al. Effect of electrical stimulation of the hypoglossal nerve on airflow mechanics in the isolated upper airway. Am Rev Respir Dis 1993;147:1144–50.

43. Oliven A, Odeh M, Schnall RP. Improved upper airway patency elicited by electrical stimulation of the hypoglossus nerves. Respiration 1996;63:213–6.

44. Eisele DW, Schwartz AR, Hari A, et al. The effects of selective nerve stimulation on upper airway airflow mechanics. Arch Otolaryngol Head Neck Surg 1995;121:1361–4.

45. Oliven A, Odeh M, Geitini L, et al. Effect of coactivation of tongue protrusor and retractor muscles on pharyngeal lumen and airflow in sleep apnea patients. J Appl Physiol 2007;103:1662–8.

46. Schwartz AR, Bennett ML, Smith PL, et al. Therapeutic electrical stimulation of the hypoglossal nerve in obstructive sleep apnea. Arch Otolaryngol Head Neck Surg 2001;127:1216–23.

47. Eastwood PR, Barnes M, Walsh JH, et al. Treating obstructive sleep apnea with hypoglossal nerve stimulation. Sleep 2011;34:1479–86.

48. Van de Heyning PH, Badr MS, Baskin JZ, et al. Implanted upper airway stimulation device for obstructive sleep apnea. Laryngoscope 2012;122:1626–33.

49. Schwartz AR, Barnes M, Hillman D, et al. Acute upper airway responses to hypoglossal nerve stimulation during sleep in obstructive sleep apnea. Am J Respir Crit Care Med 2012;185:420–6.

50. Goding GS Jr, Tesfayesus W, Kezirian EJ. Hypoglossal nerve stimulation and airway changes under fluoroscopy. Otolaryngol Head Neck Surg 2012;146:1017–22.

51. Strollo PJ Jr, Soose RJ, Maurer JT, et al. Upper-airway stimulation for obstructive sleep apnea. N Engl J Med 2014;370:139–49.

52. Woodson BT, Gillespie MB, Soose RJ, et al. Randomized controlled withdrawal study of upper airway stimulation on OSA: short-term and long-term effect. Otolaryngol Head Neck Surg 2014;151:880–7.

53. Strollo PJ Jr, Gillespie MB, Soose RJ, et al. Upper airway stimulation for obstructive sleep apnea: durability of the treatment effect at 18 months. Sleep 2015;38:1593–8.

54. Soose RJ, Woodson BT, Gillespie MB, et al. Upper airway stimulation for obstructive sleep apnea: self-reported outcomes at 24 months. J Clin Sleep Med 2015 [pii:jc-00477-14]. [Epub ahead of print].

55. Woodson BT, Soose RJ, Gillespie MB, et al. Three-year outcomes of cranial nerve stimulation for obstructive sleep apnea: the STAR trial. Otolaryngol Head Neck Surg 2015;154(1):181–8.

56. Pietzsch JB, Liu S, Garner AM, et al. Long-term cost-effectiveness of upper airway stimulation for the treatment of obstructive sleep apnea: a model-based projection based on the STAR trial. Sleep 2015;38:735–44.

57. Lee JJ, Sahu N, Rogers R, et al. Severe obstructive sleep apnea treated with combination hypoglossal nerve stimulation and oral appliance therapy. J Dental Sleep Med 2015;2(4):185–6.

Pharmacologic Approaches to the Treatment of Obstructive Sleep Apnea

David P. White, MD*

KEYWORDS

- Sleep • Apnea • Phenotypes • Loop gain • Arousal threshold • Pharmacology

KEY POINTS

- Obstructive sleep apnea is caused by various combinations of 4 phenotypic traits: pharyngeal anatomy, upper airway responsiveness, respiratory arousal threshold, and loop gain.
- There are currently no meaningful methods to influence upper airway muscle responsiveness pharmacologically. However, antagonists to potassium channels may prove to be a novel approach to accomplish this.
- Currently available hypnotics can increase the respiratory arousal threshold modestly; however, these agents have a variable effect on the severity of sleep-disordered breathing.
- Loop gain can be substantially reduced with both oxygen and acetazolamide. Both agents can lead to important decrements in the apnea-hypopnea index if the correct patients (high loop gain) are targeted.
- Although it has not been tested, combining agents to address more than 1 physiologic trait may improve efficacy compared with a single agent.

INTRODUCTION

The mainstays of therapy for obstructive sleep apnea (OSA) have always been devices or surgeries. Although neither is completely satisfactory in terms of efficacy or comfort, there have not been better options available. The concept of a pharmacologic approach to OSA treatment has always held great appeal but no agent to date has had a large enough effect size to drive substantial adoption. However, attempts continue to find the ideal or acceptable drug.

During the last 10 years, a new construct has emerged regarding the pathophysiology of OSA that may drive new thinking regarding pharmacologic therapy (**Fig. 1**). According to the new construct there are 4 primary physiologic traits that dictate who does and does not develop OSA.[1–3] These traits can vary substantially between patients, meaning that sleep apnea may develop for quite different reasons in 1 patient compared with another.[1] These traits are discussed below.

Upper Airway Anatomy or Collapsibility

For pharyngeal collapse to occur during sleep there must be some anatomic predisposition to such collapse. This is generally thought of as an anatomically small or quite collapsible airway. Possible causes of this anatomic abnormality include fat deposition in the tissue surrounding

Conflicts of Interest: Chief Medical Officer: Apnicure Inc. Consultant: Philips Respironics. Consultant: Lingua-Flex. Advisory Board: Night Balance.
Harvard Medical School, Boston, MA 02115, USA
* 4340 East Cedar Avenue, Denver, CO 80246.
E-mail address: dpwhite@partners.org

sleep.theclinics.com

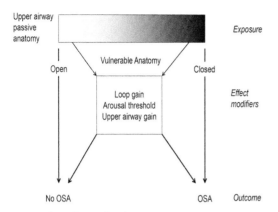

Fig. 1. The relationship between anatomy and OSA is straightforward with very favorable (no OSA) or very poor anatomy (inevitable OSA). However, the relationship of intermediate or vulnerable anatomy and OSA is modified by the other traits to lead to or protect against OSA. These other traits are effect modifiers: they modify the effect of the exposure (anatomy) on the outcome (OSA status). (*From* Owens RL, Edwards BA, Eckert DJ, et al. An integrative model of physiological traits can be used to predict obstructive sleep apnea and response to non positive airway pressure therapy. Sleep 2015;38:967; with permission.)

the airway, a reduced bony skeletal structure, or increased tonsil or adenoid size, among others. This anatomic trait is, in general, the most important single variable in dictating who does and does not develop OSA.

Upper Airway Response

In patients with an anatomically deficient airway, pharyngeal patency during wakefulness is generally maintained by increased upper airway dilator muscle activity. With sleep onset, this muscle activity decreases, yielding reduced airway size or complete collapse. This leads to hypoventilation with rising PCO_2 and increased respiratory drive, manifest as increasing intrapharyngeal negative pressure. Both airway negative pressure and increased PCO_2 can activate pharyngeal dilator muscles. If these muscles are adequately activated and are mechanically effective, they can often restore pharyngeal patency yielding rhythmic respiration and stable sleep. However, this upper airway response is quite variable between patients, with some demonstrating brisk muscle responses and others little at all. Thus, some patients can compensate during sleep for considerable anatomic deficiency, whereas others cannot.

Respiratory Arousal Threshold

In patients who require an upper airway response to restore pharyngeal patency during sleep, stable sleep must be maintained for a long enough period for the upper airway dilator muscles to be adequately recruited. In most patients, this occurs relatively slowly as PCO_2 increases and intrapharyngeal pressure becomes progressively more negative. If arousal from sleep occurs in response to the increased respiratory drive before airway patency can be adequately re-established, stable respiration during sleep cannot be achieved. Thus, a low arousal threshold to respiratory stimuli may not allow an adequate upper airway response to occur even if muscle recruitment is possible.

Loop Gain (Respiratory Control Instability)

Inherent instability in the respiratory control system can lead to a waxing and waning of respiratory drive during sleep. In individuals with an anatomic predisposition to pharyngeal collapse, as described above, airway obstruction may occur at the nadir of the waning respiratory drive yielding an obstructive apnea or hypopnea. Thus, ventilatory control instability can contribute to the development of OSA in patients with a susceptible pharyngeal airway. Loop gain is a measure of ventilatory control instability with a high loop gain indicating greater instability.

Thus, manipulation of these traits using pharmacologic agents would seem a reasonable target in the treatment of OSA.

PHARMACOLOGIC APPROACHES TO THE MANIPULATION OF OBSTRUCTIVE SLEEP APNEA TRAITS
Upper Airway Anatomy or Collapsibility

Upper airway anatomy is, almost by definition, not amenable to pharmacologic manipulation, particularly acute manipulation. The exception to this would be drugs that influence body weight, such as weight loss drugs. Changes in weight can importantly influence sleep apnea severity with substantial weight loss being a meaningful way to treat OSA.[4] Although not fully documented, it seems quite likely that weight loss primarily influences upper airway anatomy yielding a larger, less collapsible airway. It is beyond the scope of this article to address the efficacy and mechanisms of weight loss drugs. However, as appropriate, such drugs could certainly play a role in the treatment of OSA.

Upper Airway Response

The upper airway response is a restoration of a satisfactory level of ventilation primarily through the activation of upper airway dilator muscles during stable sleep. Thus, for some time now, there has been an interest in pharmacologically increasing the activity of pharyngeal dilator muscles during sleep as a method to treat OSA. The initial attempts at this were based on the proposed neural mechanisms by which loss of upper airway dilator muscle activity occurs during sleep.

Considerable literature suggests that both rapid eye movement (REM) and non-REM (NREM) sleep are associated with a substantial decrement in the firing frequencies of serotonergic (raphe) and noradrenergic (locus ceruleus) neurons.[5,6] In addition, there is clear evidence that both serotonin and noradrenaline, when applied to neurons in the hypoglossal motor nucleus (the source of neural input to the genioglossus [GG] muscle, a primary upper airway dilator muscle) depolarize the neurons and lead to increased activity.[7,8] Thus, an attempt to pharmacologically increase serotonin or noradrenaline at the motoneurons innervating upper airway dilator muscles would seem a logical approach to OSA therapy. However, during REM sleep there is additional muscarinic cholinergic inhibition of hypoglossal motoneurons,[9] which renders the neurons largely unresponsive to excitatory neurotransmitters.[8] Thus, pharmacologic agents that increase muscle activity during NREM sleep may not be effective during REM sleep and vice versa.

Serotonin

Original animal work looked promising. Veasey and colleagues[10] demonstrated that serotonin antagonists, when administered to the English bulldog, an OSA animal model, during wakefulness led to decreased upper airway dilator muscle activity and reduced airway size, suggesting an important role for serotonin in the maintenance of airway patency. In addition, Jelev and colleagues[7] demonstrated that in naturally sleeping rats the application of serotonin agonists onto the hypoglossal motor nucleus led to a substantial increase in GG electromyogram (EMG) activity during sleep, particularly during NREM sleep. However, there was little effect of serotonin antagonists on baseline GG activity during wakefulness or sleep in rats breathing room air. Finally, in a different animal model, the naturally sleeping rat with central apneas primarily during REM sleep, Carley and colleagues[11] demonstrated that a 5-hydroxytryptamine 3 (5-HT3) antagonist suppressed these central apneas. Veasey and colleagues[12] made a similar observation in the sleeping English bulldog using a different 5-HT3 antagonist. Thus, serotonin seemed to have the potential to influence sleep apnea in 2 ways: (1) direct pharyngeal dilator muscle activation primarily through 5-HT2a receptors, which should

decrease obstructive apneas, or (2) activation of peripheral 5-HT3 receptors, which leads to central apneas. This set the stage for human studies.

The human studies vary substantially in the type of serotonin agent used. In several studies selective serotonin reuptake inhibitors were administered to subjects with OSA. In these studies (using fluoxetine and paroxetine), there was a 35% to 50% reduction in obstructive apneas during NREM sleep with little effect on hypopneas and no effect on either (apneas or hypopneas) during REM sleep.[13,14] Thus, the overall apnea-hypopnea index (AHI) decreased from 57 ± 9 to 34 ± 6 in 1 study, and 36.3 ± 24.7 to 30.2 ± 18.5 in another. Stradling and colleagues[15] administered ondansetron (a 5-HT3 antagonist) to subjects with moderate to severe OSA and reported no significant change in AHI with this agent. Prasad and colleagues[16] subsequently added fluoxetine to ondansetron and, at higher doses, reported an approximately 40% decrement in AHI after 14 and 28 days of drug use. Several investigators have given the drug mirtazapine to OSA subjects. In 2 studies by Marshall and colleagues,[17] mirtazapine had no effect on AHI, whereas Carley and colleagues[18] reported a reduction in AHI from 22.3 ± 4.8 to 11.4 ± 3.6 on a higher dose of the drug (15 mg daily). However, a subsequent phase IIa trial did not support the conclusion that mirtazapine was an effective agent in the treatment of OSA. One would have to conclude from these studies that currently available drugs that influence the human serotonin system do not have a large enough effect on AHI to be useful as therapeutic agents for OSA.

Noradrenaline

Animal studies by Chan and colleagues[8] show that the alpha-adrenergic system exerts a tonic excitatory influence on the activity of upper airway motoneurons, such as the hypoglossal neurons that innervate the GG muscle. This is the case during both wakefulness and NREM sleep but not during REM sleep. Thus, the decrease in activity of noradrenergic neurons from wakeful to sleep with virtually no activity during REM sleep could explain the observed decrements in upper airway dilator muscle activity during sleep and contribute to airway collapse during sleep in OSA patients. The application of an alpha-adrenergic agonist onto hypoglossal motoneurons led to marked increases in their activity. Thus, increasing noradrenergic input to these neurons could be a viable pharmacologic path to OSA therapy.

For human trials, finding drugs that increase noradrenaline levels in the brain to investigate their effects on sleep apnea has proved difficult. Most such drugs are highly alerting, thus having a negative effect on sleep among other side effects. However, there have been several studies using protriptyline,[19–21] which is a tricyclic antidepressant whose primary mode of action is to reduce reuptake of noradrenaline, although serotonin reuptake is also inhibited to a lesser extent. The studies that used protriptyline to treat OSA consistently found that the drug reduced REM sleep time and had frequent side effects that precluded sustained use in many subjects. However, other findings were less consistent. Smith and colleagues[20] found no change is respiratory pattern during REM sleep but less apnea time during NREM sleep with less oxygen desaturation. Brownell and colleagues[19] reported reduced apnea time and desaturation during REM sleep with little change in these variables during NREM sleep. Finally, Conway and colleagues[21] observed substantial improvements in disordered breathing in some subjects and little in others with greater severity of apnea generally yielding poorer responses. Due to modest responses in most patients to protriptyline and substantial side effects, this drug is used minimally to treat OSA.

Potassium channels

The disfacilitation of hypoglossal motoneurons mediated by withdrawal of serotonergic and noradrenergic input and their direct inhibition by muscarinic cholinergic input are both modulated by increased potassium conductance. Thus, blockade of potassium channels would seem to be a potential route to increased muscle activity across all stages of sleep. This has been studied in freely behaving rats by Grace and colleagues.[22]

The application of various agents that inhibit potassium conductance directly into the hypoglossal nucleus was demonstrated to markedly increase GG muscle activity across all states (**Fig. 2**) elevating GG EMG activity to 133% to 300% of the waking level in both NREM and REM sleep.[23] This increase applied to both respiratory phasic activation and tonic expiratory activity. However, these agents were not studied using systemic application.

Because potassium channels are relatively ubiquitous in the central nervous system and their blockade generally increases neural firing, systemic application of inhibitors could lead to important side effects, the most obvious of which would be seizures. However, there is an inwardly rectifying potassium channel, Kir2.4, which seems to be expressed primarily on cranial motoneurons, including the hypoglossal motoneurons.[22] Thus, blockade of this particular channel might lead to increased upper airway muscle activation without affecting other neural processes, thus minimizing side effects. However, at this time there are no Kir2.4 antagonists. Thus, this would seem to be an ideal target for drug discovery.

Summary

Based on this information, one would have to conclude that at this time there are no available pharmacologic agents that have a large enough effect on pharyngeal dilator muscle activity to be viable OSA therapies. That being said, novel targets have been identified that, it is hoped, will lead to drug development in this important space.

Respiratory Arousal Threshold

Again, in patients with an anatomically compromised pharyngeal airway in whom the recruitment

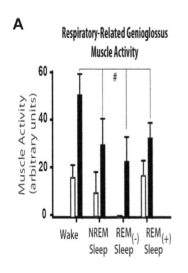

A Respiratory-Related Genioglossus Muscle Activity

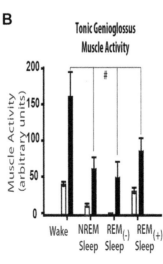

B Tonic Genioglossus Muscle Activity

Fig. 2. Microperfusion of barium into the hypoglossal motor pool restores GG muscle activity throughout sleep to waking levels. Group data (n = 6) showing the effects of barium on respiratory-related (*A*) and tonic (*B*) GG muscle activities during wakefulness, NREM, and REM sleep with ([−]) and without ([+]) muscle twitching. Hash mark indicates significant effect of barium relative to artificial cerebrospinal fluid controls independent of sleep-wake state ($P < .05$, from analysis of variance). (*From* Grace KP, Hughes SW, Horner RL. Identification of a pharmacological target for genioglossus reactivation throughout sleep. Sleep 2014;37:44; with permission.)

of pharyngeal dilator muscle activity is required to sustain airway patency during sleep, the individual must be able to stay asleep long enough for these muscle to be recruited. This process of muscle activation is generally slow because neither arterial PCO_2 nor negative intrapharyngeal airway pressure, the 2 primary drivers of upper airway muscle activity, accumulate quickly. Thus, stable sleep must be present for this to occur. This is likely the reason why sleep-disordered breathing is less severe or less commonly seen during NREM stage 3 (N3) sleep. Reaching stage N3 sleep generally requires a relatively long period of stable sleep during which muscle recruitment can occur. If muscle recruitment occurs, airway patency can be maintained and the individual can enter stage N3 sleep. If not, the individual will arouse recurrently and never reach N3 sleep.

It should also be pointed out that there is considerable variability in the level of respiratory drive required to induce arousal from sleep between individuals. Gleeson and colleagues[24] aroused normal subjects with progressive hypoxia, increasing arterial PCO_2, and the placement of a substantial inspiratory resistive load while simultaneously measuring respiratory drive (esophageal balloon). They observed that, within a given individual, the respiratory drive at the point of arousal was relatively similar regardless of the source of respiratory stimulation (hypoxia, hypercapnia, or load). On the other hand, when one individual was compared with another, the esophageal pressure (respiratory drive) at the time of arousal was vastly different (a 3-fold to 4-fold difference). This same concept has been demonstrated for patients with OSA.[25] Untreated obstructive apnea patients tend to have a considerably higher respiratory arousal threshold than normal controls. This could be attributed, at least in part, to sleep fragmentation or deprivation. However, even following months of continuous positive airway pressure (CPAP) therapy, this arousal threshold still tends to be higher than is found in the normal population. That being said, there is still considerable variability in the level of respiratory drive required to awaken an OSA patient with at least one-third of these patients having what would generally be considered a low arousal threshold even in the untreated state.[25] Thus, elevating this arousal threshold in the right patients with OSA might well be a meaningful therapeutic target.

Based on this concept, any medication that increases the level of respiratory drive required to induce arousal from sleep has the potential to buy time for upper airway muscle recruitment and possibly stabilization of airway patency. This assumes, however, that the upper airway muscles can be recruited during this time and that their activation leads to dilation or stiffening of the pharyngeal airway. If this does not occur, the apnea or hypopnea will simply be prolonged with the potential for greater hypoxia and hypercapnia. Several studies have examined the impact of hypnotic medications on the respiratory arousal threshold. Eckert and colleagues,[26,27] in separate studies, examined the influence of eszopiclone (3 mg) and trazodone (100 mg) on epiglottic pressure (a measure of respiratory drive) at the point of arousal. Both drugs were found to increase the level of epiglottic pressure required to induce arousal. Ezopiclone[27] increased this measure from -14.0 to -18.0 cm H_2O and trazodone[26] from -11.5 to -15.3 cm H_2O. Eikermann and colleagues[28] also reported that pentobarbital increased the time to arousal induced by progressive decrements in CPAP pressure from the holding pressure (pressure required to prevent flow limitation during sleep). The actual mask pressure at the point of arousal was also lower with pentobarbital compared with placebo. Thus, the arousal threshold in response to respiratory stimuli can be manipulated pharmacologically although the effect was relatively modest.

The obvious question this raises is whether these changes in respiratory arousal threshold influenced the severity of sleep-disordered breathing. Most studies that assessed the effect of hypnotics on apnea severity did not phenotype the subjects. Thus, they did not know whether the subjects being treated had a low or high arousal threshold. They also did not know the other phenotypic traits. With that in mind, studies of eszopiclone,[29] nitrazepam,[30] ramelteon,[31] temazepam,[32] and zopiclone[33] when administered to either OSA subjects or subjects with the upper airway resistance syndrome did not lead to substantial decrements in the apnea index or the AHI. Most improved sleep quality but systematic changes in sleep-disordered breathing were not observed. That being said, in several studies, when individual data were provided, substantial decrements in AHI were observed in some of the subjects, whereas little change was observed in others. This was clearly the case with eszopiclone[29] and nitrazepam[30] but not temazepam.[32] Whether the responding subjects had a low arousal threshold and the nonresponding ones a high threshold is unclear. Other phenotypic traits could also have driven this variable response. Finally, night to night variability in AHI may also have contributed.

Several studies did measure arousal threshold or all of the phenotypic traits before the administration of the hypnotic. Eckert and colleagues[27] found that eszopiclone reduced the AHI from 31 to 24 in 17 OSA patients with broad variability in arousal threshold. However, when the 8 subjects with a low arousal threshold (greater than -15 cm H_2O epiglottic pressure at arousal) were evaluated, their AHI decreased from 25 to 14, ($P<.01$), with no overall change in the AHI in the subjects with a higher (more negative) arousal threshold ($P = .52$) (**Fig. 3**). Thus, in this study, arousal threshold did strongly influence who did and did not respond to the hypnotic. However, when Eckert and colleagues[26] studied trazodone, the results were quite different. Trazodone was administered to 7 subjects, all of whom had a low arousal threshold (greater than -15 cm H_2O). Trazodone increased the arousal threshold by $32 \pm 6\%$ but had no effect on AHI (39 ± 12 vs 39 ± 11, $P = .94$), critical pressure (Pcrit; a measure of upper airway collapsibility), GG muscle activity or responsiveness. The explanation for this poor response is unclear but may be related to the high Pcrit (highly collapsible airway) of many of these subjects. Five of the 7 subjects had a Pcrit greater than 0 cm H_2O on trazodone and one a Pcrit of -0.3 cm H_2O. The 1 patient with modest collapsibility (Pcrit of -4.0 cm H_2O) demonstrated a reduction in AHI from 31 to 20 on trazodone.

Summary

One would have to conclude from these data that hypnotics can increase the respiratory arousal threshold, although the increments are somewhat modest using the drugs tested to date. However, these increments in respiratory arousal threshold do not systematically improve sleep-disordered breathing. The data suggest that patients with a lower arousal threshold may respond better than those with a higher threshold although other phenotypic traits likely influence this responsiveness. One could speculate that the patients most likely to respond to a hypnotic have a low arousal threshold, not terribly abnormal upper airway anatomy or collapsibility, and a good upper airway response (muscle activation). However, this hypothesis will require verification.

Loop Gain (Ventilatory Control Instability)

Loop gain is an engineering term that describes the gain of any system controlled by feedback loops. Respiratory control is certainly such a system designed primarily to control arterial PCO_2. If PCO_2 increases, ventilation increases, and if PCO_2 decreases, so will ventilation. A high respiratory loop gain indicates a control system that responds substantially to even small changes in arterial PCO_2. A respiratory control system with a high loop gain has the propensity to be unstable with a waxing and waning of ventilatory drive and ventilation. As stated previously, at the nadir of such waxing and waning of ventilator drive, the respiratory output to the upper airway muscles can be minimal, leading to pharyngeal collapse in an individual with an anatomically predisposed airway. Thus, a high loop gain can contribute to the development of OSA.

There are 2 primary components to respiratory loop gain: plant gain and control gain. The plant consists of the lungs and respiratory muscles and its gain is simply the relationship between ventilation and arterial PCO_2 (ie, if one breathes more or less, how much is PCO_2 affected?). The controller gain is driven by the carbon dioxide

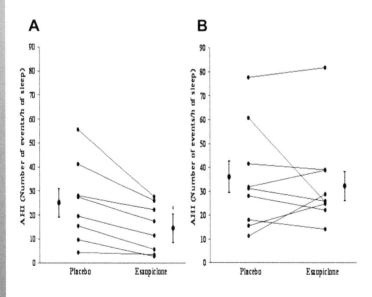

Fig. 3. AHI scatter plots during the placebo and eszopiclone condition in (*A*) the patients with (n = 8) and (*B*) the patients without (n = 9) a low respiratory arousal threshold (between 0 and -15 cm H_2O). Mean $\pm$ standard error of the mean values are presented adjacent to each condition. Significant difference compared with placebo (*asterisk*). (*From* Eckert DJ, Owens RL, Kehlmann GB, et al. Eszopiclone increases the respiratory arousal threshold and lowers the AHI in obstructive sleep apnea patients with a low arousal threshold. Clin Sci (Lond) 2011;120:510; with permission.)

sensors located in the carotid body and brainstem (retrotrapezoid nucleus). The gain of the controller is simply the hypercapnic ventilator response (ie, as PCO_2 increases, how much does ventilation increase?). The controller gain is quite variable between individuals and is the main driver of loop gain in most people.

Loop gain is generally unitless and is quantified by measuring a ventilator response to a ventilator disturbance: Loop gain = ventilatory response/ventilatory disturbance. Thus, a large response to a small disturbance yields a high loop gain. Although not commonly done and certainly not in a clinical setting, loop gain be measured in several ways, the simplest of which is to simply create a ventilatory disturbance and measure the response.[2,3] However, a full description of this and other techniques is beyond the scope of this article.

If loop gain is an important determinant of OSA, it would certainly be an exciting pharmacologic target as there are several ways to fairly easily reduce loop gain. Its importance is suggested by the work of Younes and colleagues[34] who found that subjects with severe OSA had a higher loop gain than subjects with less severe disease. However, most studies directly comparing loop gain in OSA subjects versus controls have not reported systematic differences.[1] That being said, Eckert and colleagues[1] reported that in OSA subjects with only a mildly collapsible upper airway, loop gain was 50% higher than in subjects with a more collapsible airway. Thus, in certain OSA patients, a high loop gain may be an important determinant of disease.

Oxygen

One of the easiest ways to lower loop gain is the administration of oxygen, which reduces responsiveness to PCO_2 at both the carotid body and the central chemoreceptor. This effect of oxygen on loop gain has been clearly demonstrated by Edwards and colleagues,[35] who also found that the other phenotypic traits were not affected by oxygen. Oxygen was explored as a form of therapy for OSA in the early days after the disorder was originally described.[36,37] In most such studies oxygen did not lead to an important decrement in the frequency of sleep-disordered breathing when the entire cohort of OSA subjects was examined. However, in most such studies 20% to 30% of subjects demonstrated an important decrement in AHI with oxygen administration.[36,37] One can speculate that the oxygen responders had a high loop gain and other phenotypic traits that made them amenable to such therapy, whereas the other subjects did not.

Wellman and colleagues[38] systematically measured loop gain on and off oxygen in a group of OSA subjects and determined the effect of oxygen on AHI in these subjects. In subjects with a high loop gain, oxygen substantially lowered loop gain (0.60 ± 0.18 to 0.34 ± 0.04) and reduced the AHI by 53% (**Fig. 4**). In subjects with a low loop gain, oxygen had little effect on loop gain and the AHI decreased by only 8%. Thus, oxygen can importantly affect the severity of sleep-disordered breathing if the phenotypically correct patients (high loop gain) are selected for therapy.

Acetazolamide

Although acetazolamide has been widely studied as a therapy for central sleep apnea both in patients with and without congestive heart failure, it has not been commonly evaluated in subjects with OSA. However, Edwards and colleagues[39] did study 13 subjects with OSA both on and off acetazolamide, in addition to defining the phenotypic traits of these subjects under both conditions. Acetazolamide substantially reduced the loop gain in 12 of the 13 subjects (median loop gain fell from 3.4 to 2.0) but had little effect on the other 3 traits. In addition, the drug led to a substantial reduction in sleep-disordered breathing with the NREM median AHI decreasing from 50 to 24 (**Fig. 5**). This was a 51% reduction. In addition, the REM AHI decreased by 35%. Thus, in this group of patients, acetazolamide led to an

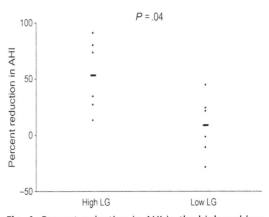

Fig. 4. Percent reduction in AHI in the high and low loop gain (LG) groups. Oxygen reduced the AHI from 63 ± 34 episodes/h to 34 ± 30 episodes/h in the high LG group ($53 \pm 33\%$ reduction) and from 44 ± 34 episodes/h to 37 ± 28 episodes/h in the low LG group ($8 \pm 27\%$ reduction). Mean value for each group noted with black bar. (*From* Wellman A, Malhotra A, Jordan AS, et al. Effect of oxygen in obstructive sleep apnea: role of loop gain. Respir Physiol Neurobiol 2008;162:147; with permission.)

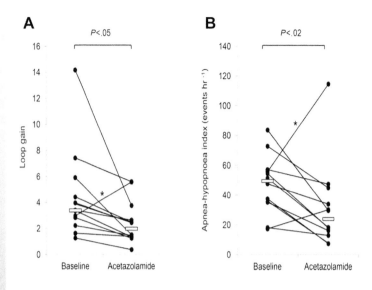

Fig. 5. Individual effects of acetazolamide on LG and the severity of sleep-disordered breathing. (*A*) Individual data comparing steady-state LG during baseline and acetazolamide conditions. Note that the steady-state LG was reduced in all but 1 subject. (*B*) Acetazolamide significantly reduced the median AHI from 49.6 (35.5–56.6) to 24.1 (12.9–42.3) events per hour, during supine NREM sleep. Median values for each condition are indicated by the solid white bars. Note that the 1 subject whose LG doubled with acetazolamide also exhibited a similar rise in AHI (*asterisk*). (*From* Edwards BA, Sands SA, Eckert DJ, et al. Acetazolamide improves loop gain but not the other physiological traits causing obstructive sleep apnoea. J Physiol 2012;590:1206; with permission.)

important decrement in the frequency of disordered breathing that is likely attributable to the reduced loop gain.

Summary

From the relatively small studies described, one could draw several conclusions. First, loop gain is quite variable in patients with OSA with higher loop gains being associated with more severe apnea. Second, loop gain can be substantially manipulated with either oxygen or acetazolamide. Finally, decrements in loop gain commonly lead to a reduction in the frequency of sleep-disordered breathing.

HISTORICAL PHARMACOLOGIC APPROACHES UNRELATED TO OBSTRUCTIVE SLEEP APNEA TRAITS

During the last 3 to 4 decades, attempts to treat OSA with several pharmacologic agents have been attempted. None of these studies yielded particularly encouraging results or certainly not results adequate to drive any adoption. Examples include ventilator stimulants, such as progesterone[40]; agents to increase cholinergic tone, such as donepezil[41]; and a glutamate antagonist.[42] Thus, currently, medications are not commonly used to treat sleep apnea.

SUMMARY

1. OSA is caused by various combinations of 4 phenotypic traits: pharyngeal anatomy, upper airway responsiveness, respiratory arousal threshold, and loop gain.

2. There are currently no meaningful methods to influence upper airway muscle responsiveness pharmacologically. However, antagonists to potassium channels may prove to be a novel approach to accomplish this.

3. Currently available hypnotics can increase the respiratory arousal threshold modestly; however, these agents have a variable effect on the severity of sleep-disordered breathing.

4. Loop gain can be substantially reduced with oxygen and acetazolamide. Both agents can lead to important decrements in AHI if the correct patients (high loop gain) are targeted.

5. Although it has not been tested, combining agents to address more than a single physiologic trait may well improve efficacy compared with a single agent.

REFERENCES

1. Eckert DJ, White DP, Jordan AS, et al. Defining phenotypic causes of obstructive sleep apnea. Identification of novel therapeutic targets. Am J Respir Crit Care Med 2013;188:996–1004.

2. Wellman A, Eckert DJ, Jordan AS, et al. A method for measuring and modeling the physiological traits causing obstructive sleep apnea. J Appl Physiol 2011;110:1627–37.

3. Wellman A, Edwards BA, Sands SA, et al. A simplified method for determining phenotypic traits in patients with obstructive sleep apnea. J Appl Physiol 2013;114:911–22.

4. Newman AB, Foster G, Givelber R, et al. Progression and regression of sleep-disordered breathing with changes in weight: the Sleep Heart Health Study. Arch Intern Med 2005;165:2408–13.

5. Trulson ME, Jacobs BL. Raphe unit activity in freely moving cats: correlation with level of behavioral arousal. Brain Res 1979;163:135–50.

6. Saper CB, Scammell TE, Lu J. Hypothalamic regulation of sleep and circadian rhythms. Nature 2005; 437:1257–63.

7. Jelev A, Sood S, Liu H, et al. Microdialysis perfusion of 5-HT into hypoglossal motor nucleus differentially modulates genioglossus activity across natural sleep-wake states in rats. J Physiol 2001;532:467–81.

8. Chan E, Steenland HW, Liu H, et al. Endogenous excitatory drive modulating respiratory muscle activity across sleep-wake states. Am J Respir Crit Care Med 2006;174:1264–73.

9. Grace KP, Hughes SW, Horner RL. Identification of the mechanism mediating genioglossus muscle suppression in REM sleep. Am J Respir Crit Care Med 2013;187:311–9.

10. Veasey SC, Panckeri KA, Hoffman EA, et al. The effects of serotonin antagonists in an animal model of sleep-disordered breathing. Am J Respir Crit Care Med 1996;153:776–86.

11. Carley DW, Depoortere H, Radulovacki M. R-zacopride, a 5-HT3 antagonist/5-HT4 agonist, reduces sleep apneas in rats. Pharmacol Biochem Behav 2001;69:283–9.

12. Veasey SC, Chachkes J, Fenik P, et al. The effects of ondansetron on sleep-disordered breathing in the English bulldog. Sleep 2001;24:155–60.

13. Hanzel DA, Proia NG, Hudgel DW. Response of obstructive sleep apnea to fluoxetine and protriptyline. Chest 1991;100:416–21.

14. Kraiczi H, Hedner J, Dahlöf P, et al. Effect of serotonin uptake inhibition on breathing during sleep and daytime symptoms in obstructive sleep apnea. Sleep 1999;22:61–7.

15. Stradling J, Smith D, Radulovacki M, et al. Effect of ondansetron on moderate obstructive sleep apnoea, a single night, placebo-controlled trial. J Sleep Res 2003;12:169–70.

16. Prasad B, Radulovacki M, Olopade C, et al. Prospective trial of efficacy and safety of ondansetron and fluoxetine in patients with obstructive sleep apnea syndrome. Sleep 2010;33:982–9.

17. Marshall NS, Yee BJ, Desai AV, et al. Two randomized placebo-controlled trials to evaluate the efficacy and tolerability of mirtazapine for the treatment of obstructive sleep apnea. Sleep 2008;3:824–31.

18. Carley DW, Olopade C, Ruigt GS, et al. Efficacy of mirtazapine in obstructive sleep apnea syndrome. Sleep 2007;30:35–41.

19. Brownell LG, Perez-Padilla R, West P, et al. The role of protriptyline in obstructive sleep apnea. Bull Eur Physiopathol Respir 1983;19:621–4.

20. Smith PL, Haponik EF, Allen RP, et al. The effects of protriptyline in sleep-disordered breathing. Am Rev Respir Dis 1983;127:8–13.

21. Conway WA, Zorick F, Piccione P, et al. Protriptyline in the treatment of sleep apnoea. Thorax 1982;37: 49–53.

22. Grace KP, Hughes SW, Shahabi S, et al. K+ channel modulation causes genioglossus inhibition in REM sleep and is a strategy for reactivation. Respir Physiol Neurobiol 2013;188:277–88.

23. Grace KP, Hughes SW, Horner RL. Identification of a pharmacological target for genioglossus reactivation throughout sleep. Sleep 2014;37:41–50.

24. Gleeson K, Zwillich CW, White DP. The influence of increasing ventilatory effort on arousal from sleep. Am Rev Respir Dis 1990;142:295–300.

25. Eckert DJ, Younes MK. Arousal from sleep: implications for obstructive sleep apnea pathogenesis and treatment. J Appl Physiol 2014;116:302–13.

26. Eckert DJ, Malhotra A, Wellman A, et al. Trazodone increases the respiratory arousal threshold in patients with obstructive sleep apnea and a low arousal threshold. Sleep 2014;37:811–9.

27. Eckert DJ, Owens RL, Kehlmann GB, et al. Eszopiclone increases the respiratory arousal threshold and lowers the apnoea/hypopnoea index in obstructive sleep apnoea patients with a low arousal threshold. Clin Sci (Lond) 2011;120:505–14.

28. Eikermann M, Eckert DJ, Chamberlin NL, et al. Effects of pentobarbital on upper airway patency during sleep. Eur Respir J 2010;36:569–76.

29. Rosenberg R, Roach JM, Scharf M, et al. A pilot study evaluating acute use of eszopiclone in patients with mild to moderate obstructive sleep apnea syndrome. Sleep Med 2007;8:464–70.

30. Höijer U, Hedner J, Ejnell H, et al. Nitrazepam in patients with sleep apnoea: a double-blind placebo-controlled study. Eur Respir J 1994;7:2011–5.

31. Kryger M, Roth T, Wang-Weigand S, et al. The effects of ramelteon on respiration during sleep in subjects with moderate to severe chronic obstructive pulmonary disease. Sleep Breath 2009;13:79–84.

32. Wang D, Marshall NS, Duffin J, et al. Phenotyping interindividual variability in obstructive sleep apnoea response to temazepam using ventilatory chemoreflexes during wakefulness. J Sleep Res 2011;20: 526–32.

33. Lofaso F, Goldenberg F, Thebault C, et al. Effect of zopiclone on sleep, night-time ventilation, and daytime vigilance in upper airway resistance syndrome. Eur Respir J 1997;10:2573–7.

34. Younes M, Ostrowski M, Thompson W, et al. Chemical control stability in patients with obstructive sleep apnea. Am J Respir Crit Care Med 2001;163:1181–90.

35. Edwards BA, Sands SA, Owens RL, et al. Effects of hyperoxia and hypoxia on the physiological traits responsible for obstructive sleep apnea. J Physiol 2014;592:4523–35.

36. Kearley R, Wynne JW, Block AJ, et al. The effect of low flow oxygen on sleep-disordered breathing and oxygen desaturation. A study of patients with chronic obstructive lung disease. Chest 1980;78: 682–5.

37. Smith PL, Haponik EF, Bleecker ER. The effects of oxygen in patients with sleep apnea. Am Rev Respir Dis 1984;130:958–63.

38. Wellman A, Malhotra A, Jordan AS, et al. Effect of oxygen in obstructive sleep apnea: role of loop gain. Respir Physiol Neurobiol 2008;162:144–51.

39. Edwards BA, Sands SA, Eckert DJ, et al. Acetazolamide improves loop gain but not the other physiological traits causing obstructive sleep apnoea. J Physiol 2012;590:1199–2111.

40. Rajagopal KR, Abbrecht PH, Jabbari B. Effects of medroxyprogesterone acetate in obstructive sleep apnea. Chest 1986;90:815–21.

41. Moraes W, Poyares D, Sukys-Claudino L, et al. Donepezil improves obstructive sleep apnea in Alzheimer disease: a double-blind, placebo-controlled study. Chest 2008;133:677–83.

42. Hedner J, Grunstein R, Eriksson B, et al. A double-blind, randomized trial of sabeluzole–a putative glutamate antagonist–in obstructive sleep apnea. Sleep 1996;19:287–9.

The Challenges of Precision Medicine in Obstructive Sleep Apnea

Abdelnaby Khalyfa, PhD, Alex Gileles-Hillel, MD,
David Gozal, MD, MBA*

KEYWORDS

- Biomarkers • Sleep apnea • Gene arrays • Proteomics • Epigenetics

KEY POINTS

- Obstructive sleep apnea (OSA) is highly prevalent, but its diagnosis requires an onerous and not always readily available approach.
- OSA is associated with a very variable phenotype and with increased risk for end-organ morbidities that are difficult to detect unless specifically sought out.
- Biomarkers for OSA are unlikely to perform well if identified in isolation, and therefore, biomarker signatures are preferable.
- Biomarker signatures should explore (i) diagnostic approaches; (ii) morbidity; (iii) treatment monitoring and outcomes.

SLEEP-DISORDERED BREATHING AND OBSTRUCTIVE SLEEP APNEA

Sleep is an essential biological function with major roles in energy, recovery, conservation, and survival. Good quality of sleep is therefore critical for good health and overall quality of life. Nevertheless, millions of people do not get enough sleep, and many suffer from lack of sleep. Furthermore, sleep disorders are extremely common and lead to substantial morbidity, high health care costs, and reduced quality of life. Disrupted sleep in general, and more particularly, the highly prevalent condition of obstructive sleep apnea (OSA) have emerged as major risk factors for other diseases, such as obesity, high blood pressure, cardiovascular and metabolic disease, cognitive dysfunction, and depression.[1] Untreated patients with OSA suffer up to a 7-fold increased risk of motor vehicle collisions. The negative impacts of sleep apnea and sleepiness on work performance are also being increasingly recognized. Multiple studies have also demonstrated that treatment of OSA is an extremely cost-effective use of health care resources.[2–4]

Sleep patterns and duration vary both among species and within species,[5] and such variability may be due to in part to segregating genetic variation,[6] implying that sleep and risk factors for sleep disorders are at least partly under genetic control. However, the genes accounting for genetic variation in sleep are not known. Similarly, the genes underlying the risk for OSA have only been partially explored, and to date, in-depth exploration of the contribution and mechanisms underlying the role of selected genes that emerged from genome wide scans are lacking.[7–13]

Disclosure Statement: No conflicts of interest to declare.
Funding Sources: D. Gozal is supported by the Herbert T. Abelson Endowed Chair in Pediatrics.
Section of Pediatric Sleep Medicine, Department of Pediatrics, Pritzker School of Medicine, Biological Sciences Division, The University of Chicago, Chicago, IL, USA
* Corresponding author. Department of Pediatrics, Pritzker School of Medicine, The University of Chicago, KCBD, Room 4100, 900 East 57th Street, Mailbox 4, Chicago, IL 60637-1470.
E-mail address: dgozal@uchicago.edu

sleep.theclinics.com

Based on the aforementioned genetic studies, it has been suggested that OSA is unlikely to represent a simple condition associated with a few genes or proteins; instead, it is likely a manifestation of multiple interconnected pathways and numerous molecular abnormalities.[14] In addition, OSA is a strong risk factor for many other diseases, and conversely, many other diseases increase the risk of OSA. For example, OSA is associated with inflammatory states and oxidative stress,[15–17] and obesity, one of the prominent risk factors for OSA, coenhances the presence other morbidities, such as insulin resistance, hypertension, cardiovascular disease, and neurocognitive dysfunction[18–21] (Fig. 1).

PEDIATRIC OBSTRUCTIVE SLEEP APNEA

Similar to adults, pediatric obstructive sleep apnea (P-OSA) is characterized by episodic events associated with either partial or complete obstruction of the airway during sleep, leading to intermittent oxygen desaturations, recurrent and often sustained increases in carbon dioxide, increases in the magnitude of intrathoracic inspiratory pressures, and in many instances, the occurrence of arousals from sleep with resultant sleep fragmentation.[22] P-OSA is a common condition affecting 2% to 4% of the childhood population,[23] and similar to adult patients, can result in significant end-organ morbidities, particularly involving the central nervous, cardiovascular, and metabolic systems.[22,24–28] These end-organ morbidities not only can be immediate but also can affect patients long term,[29] while also incurring higher health care costs, thereby further indicating the pressing need for timely diagnosis and treatment.[30,31]

However, even a thorough clinical history and physical examination are remarkably poor at differentiating between OSA and habitual primary snoring,[32] such that current diagnostic approaches require implementation of in-laboratory or home-based polysomnography (PSG) or similar diagnostic multichannel recording tests.[33–37] Indeed, PSG is labor intensive, inconvenient, and expensive, resulting in long waiting periods and unnecessary delays in diagnosis and treatment. From this perspective, the identification of surrogate biomarkers that reliably diagnose OSA would substantially overcome these problems and enable early detection and intervention for this important medical problem.

ADULT OBSTRUCTIVE SLEEP APNEA

Similar to the pediatric age range, the prevalence of adult obstructive sleep apnea (A-OSA) is high and rather variable (4% to 15%), with major contributions of age, gender, and ethnicity.[38,39] OSA has emerged in the last decades as a major public health issue with society-wide adverse consequences involving car- or work-related accidents, cognitive and behavioral deficits impairing work performance, in addition to increasing the risk cardiovascular and metabolic dysfunction.[40] More recent studies further suggest that there is a link between sleep apnea and diabetes, depression, as well as cancer,[41–43] such that OSA accounts either directly or via its associated morbidities for a substantial proportion of all medical-related costs.[44,45]

TREATMENT OF OBSTRUCTIVE SLEEP APNEA

In adults, continuous positive airway pressure (CPAP) is the gold-standard treatment for patients with symptomatic OSA. CPAP has few major side effects, and for most patients, an initial trial with CPAP is recommended. Some patients have transformative benefits from CPAP,[46,47] but new therapies or improvements in existing therapies for OSA are needed in view of the large number

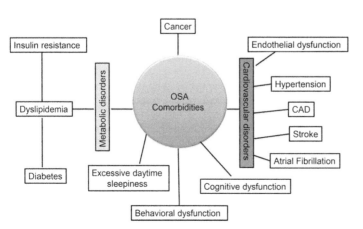

Fig. 1. The multifaceted aspects of OSA. CAD, coronary artery disease.

of patients who are intolerant or nonadherent of CPAP.[46,48] Although CPAP therapy is highly efficacious when used throughout the duration of sleep, its benefits are limited by the variable adherence, with as many as 25% of patients stopping CPAP use after 1 year. It should be emphasized that all of OSA treatments, including CPAP, upper-airway surgery, weight loss, and oral appliances, require repeated PSG monitoring for titration or follow-up.[49] Thus, the availability of biomarkers that are indicative of favorable response to therapy would be highly desirable.

In children, adenotonsillar hypertrophy has been recognized as the major pathophysiologic contributor of P-OSA and has been customarily managed by surgical removal of enlarged adenoids and tonsils with overall significant improvements, albeit not necessarily complete resolution being reported for all treated patients with OSA.[50,51] Indeed, surgical adenotonsillectomy (T&A) for OSA has come under scrutiny, particularly regarding the possibility that a significant proportion of the polysomnographic abnormalities associated with OSA may not normalize after surgery, thereby prompting the need for development of nonsurgical therapeutic alternatives.[52] Because, as stated above, the diagnosis of OSA is virtually impossible while relying on clinical tools, the detection of those children with residual OSA after T&A is even less likely without a repeat PSG, indicating the need for potential biomarkers in this context.

Thus, whether when dealing with A-OSA or P-OSA, availability of straightforward biomarker-based tools for diagnosis, monitoring of treatment success and adherence, and accurate detection of those individuals at risk for developing complication from OSA constitute highly desirable goals.

THE LONG AND COMPLEX ROAD TO BIOMARKER DISCOVERY AND IMPLEMENTATION

The definition of a biomarker has gone through multiple evolutionary perspectives. Nowadays, a biomarker would be viewed as a "biological molecule found in blood, other body fluids, or tissues that is a sign of normal or abnormal processes or of a condition or disease"[53] (**Fig. 2**). In the context of OSA, 3 major areas of investigation focused on biomarkers have emerged as essential for the field and will undoubtedly require substantial discovery and validation efforts: (i) diagnostic biomarkers: a panel of biological candidates that reliably discriminates between individuals with and without OSA; (ii) morbidity biomarkers: a panel of readily measurable biological products that reliably discerns among patients with OSA by detecting those at risk for developing or already present end-organ morbidities; (iii) treatment adherence/outcomes: biological approaches that identify those patients under higher risk of residual OSA or individuals with a differential response to treatment that places them at risk for morbidity.

There are 2 general approaches that have been used to investigate the aforementioned issues in OSA: candidate-based approaches (biased) and "omics" screens (unbiased) (**Fig. 3**). Candidate-based genetic studies, for example, compare the frequency of gene variants thought to relate to disease susceptibility in groups with and without OSA. On the other hand, high-throughput platforms enabling the investigation of specific domains of the cell/tissue machinery, such as mass spectrometry, microarrays, and next generation sequencing, are aimed at the universal

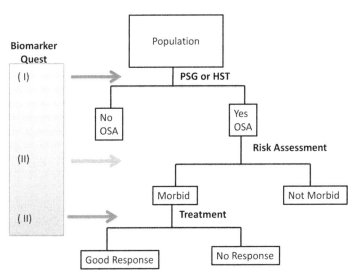

Fig. 2. Approaches to discovery and implementation of putative biomarker signatures in the context of diagnosis and management of OSA. HST, home sleep testing.

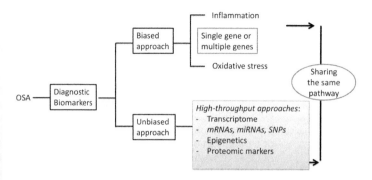

Fig. 3. Approaches to biomarker discovery predicated on a priori biased or unbiased approaches.

detection of genes (genomics), messenger RNA (mRNA) (transcriptomics), proteins (proteomics), and epigenetics in a specific biological sample, as illustrated in **Fig. 4**A.

The publication of the full human genome sequence in 2003 by the International Human Genome Sequencing Consortium is a crucial milestone in the history of genetic research, which has paved the way for "genome" and "genomics" research and initiated the so-called postgenomic area in biomedical research.[54] Consequently, the research focus has moved beyond the genome to the role of genes, a much more challenging task, including the understanding of gene transcriptional regulation, the biochemical functions of all the gene products and their interactions, and learning how they influence the chemicals that control cellular biochemistry and metabolism. In the last decade, the application of "omics" techniques has allowed the detection of small changes in protein or metabolic profiles in human samples, such as tissue, plasma, saliva, cerebrospinal fluid, and urine, providing a "signature" of human diseases (**Fig. 4**B).

The enormous amounts of data generated by "omics" have not only required the development of unique tools for analysis but also further pointed to the need for parallel and cooperative involvement of biostatisticians and bioinformaticians. Understanding the genetic basis of complex traits is and will continue to be an ongoing quest for many researchers in medicine, and integration of data originating from multiple levels of biological systems—that is, DNA sequence data,[55] RNA expression levels,[56] methylation patterns,[57] other epigenetic markers,[58] proteomics,[59] and metabolomics,[1,60] will further enhance the capability to understand the system complexities, but should also enable prediction of individual variants, leading to the desired personalized precision (see **Fig. 4**B). Even if the authors are still distant from achieving such goals, nothing is lost in the process of implementing efforts aimed at

identifying genes and pathways associated with OSA, which can expand the understanding of the risk factors for the disease as well as provide new avenues for potential treatment (see **Fig. 3**). Most sleep disorders, including OSA, are caused by complex interactions between genes and the environment, such that the authors need to focus on the genes that predetermine susceptibility to the disease as well as identify the effects of hypoxia, hypercapnia, increased respiratory efforts, and sleep fragmentation on the expression of candidate genes.[14,61]

TRANSCRIPTOMICS

Transcriptomic approaches investigate mRNA changes under a variety of biological conditions. Although much has been learned of the pathophysiology and consequences of OSA, the mechanisms and specific genes linked with such processes are not yet fully delineated.

Previous analysis of mRNA from whole blood samples in OSA patients revealed changes in several genes involved in modulation of reactive oxygen species, including heme oxygenase 1, superoxide dismutase 1 and 2, catalase, and genes involved in cell growth, proliferation, and cell-cycle control.[62] However, whether assessment of gene expression patterns in the blood constitutes a proper surrogate for the gene expression in the diseased tissues is debatable. To this effect, comparison of the peripheral blood transcriptome with genes expressed in 9 different human tissue types revealed that expression of more than 80% was identical among any given tissue, although the use of peripheral gene expression as a substitute for those in the central nervous system has been questioned.[63,64]

Using transcriptomic analyses of peripheral white blood cells in children with OSA has shown promising findings.[61,65] Assessment of 20 children with OSA and matched controls identified 36 uniquely different mRNAs.[61] Implementation of

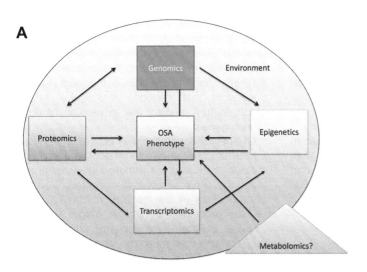

A

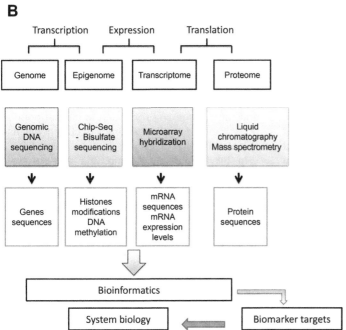

B

Fig. 4. Potential technologies aimed at biomarker discovery in the context of OSA (*A*) and downstream pipeline (*B*).

hierarchical clustering analytics further allowed for relatively accurate identification of OSA and non-OSA children.[66] To better understand potential pathways that might be implicated in biological processes affected among children with OSA, the authors imported the differentially expressed genes onto relevant bioinformatics software and identified multiple pathways particularly encompassing the inflammatory response, cell survival, cell proliferation, and differentiation pathways. Of these, the highest number of interactions in these pathways was within the inflammatory network, indicating and confirming for the first time the unique nature of OSA as a putative low-grade systemic inflammatory disease.[67,68]

In another set of studies, the authors explored using genome-wide expression analysis for the expression patterns in circulating leukocytes of children with habitual snoring and a normal sleep study and nonsnoring matched controls.[65] Gene set enrichment analysis that identified over-representation of curated pathways instead of individual genes revealed 6 broadly distinct pathways that encompassed both metabolic and inflammation-related functions. Thus, even at the low end of the spectrum of severity of sleep-disordered breathing, there appears to be evidence of perturbations encompassing some of the end-organ morbidities described for OSA in children.

Because P-OSA is commonly caused by enlarged tonsils and adenoids impinging on the patency of the upper airway during sleep, the authors performed genome-wide transcriptional profiling of tonsillar tissues obtained from children with and without OSA and outlined a computational framework to identify novel candidate targets regulating adenotonsillar hypertrophy.[69] Many of these gene candidates were involved in inflammation signaling (eg, IL1B, IL1A, IL1F6, IL6, CCL19) and regulation (eg, JUNB, FOS), and tissue growth and remodeling (eg, TGFB1, TGFB2, HBEGF, CTGF, FN1). However, 2 protein phosphatases, namely dual-specificity phosphatase 1 and phosphoserine phosphatase, were among the statistically significant network genes, and in vitro verification of their functional roles illustrated their ability to induce proliferative responses of upper airway lymphadenoid tissues, thus providing putative nonsurgical therapeutic targets.[69]

Microarray-based technologies have also been used to identify differentially expressed genes in Asian adult patients with OSA.[70] These investigators examined peripheral blood mononuclear cells (PBMC) and suggested that the genes ADAM29, FLRT2, and SLC18A3 could be included as part of a routine screen to help identify individuals at risk of severe OSA in Asian populations. In yet another study in the United States, gene network approaches were applied to visceral fat tissues (visceral fat biopsies were obtained intraoperatively), and the investigators identified several pathways intricately involved in the regulation of adipocyte metabolism and inflammation that may be important modulators of metabolic disturbances associated with OSA.[71]

These preliminary studies support the assumption that transcriptomic approaches not only will provide insights into putative mechanisms underlying the effects of end-organ morbidities in OSA but also may potentially be used to define unique clinical phenotypes[72–75] and potentially be of value in diagnostic screening approaches.

CIRCULATING MICRORNA

MicroRNAs (miRNAs) are short noncoding (19–23 nucleotides) regulatory RNAs that modulate biological homeostasis by controlling gene expression through mRNA targeting and translational repression.[76] Since their discovery in the 1990s, they have gained tremendous interest because of their potential functional roles in regulating gene expression. The presence of circulating miRNAs in plasma suggests that miRNAs may fulfill important biological functions outside of their corresponding cell sources in both physiologic and pathologic conditions and serve as potential biomarkers for disease states.[77] miRNAs can act either on target mRNA transcripts or by first regulating intermediate components such as transcripts that encode transcription factors, which, in turn, control the expression of downstream genes.

Of note, although the miRNAs found in plasma and serum are thought to reflect the extrusion of miRNAs from relevant remote tissues or organs, they may serve as disease indicators[78] and are also involved in the regulation of several key cellular processes in remote target cells that include cellular development, differentiation, proliferation, cell death, and metabolism.[79] Because miRNAs can be readily detected in various body fluids,[80,81] they have been advanced as useful biomarker candidates for the diagnosis and characterization of systemic diseases,[82] including type 2 diabetes mellitus,[83] hypertension,[84] obesity,[85] and cardiovascular disease.[86,87] Peripheral blood miRNAs, including miRNAs expressed by PBMC, as well as extracellular/circulating miRNAs may thus provide an easy and rapid screening approach in clinical populations[88] and add to the accuracy of current disease risk stratification criteria.

In this contextual setting, the authors have recently explored the presence of a selective signature in children with endothelial dysfunction and found that 3 specific miRNAs, namely hsa-miR-125a-5p, hsa-miR-342-3p, and hsa-miR-365b-3p, are potential biomarkers of children at risk for future cardiovascular disease.[89]

In a cohort of patients with resistant hypertension suffering from OSA, the authors identified plasma miRNA profiles that predict blood pressure responses to CPAP treatment.[90] It has now been quite well established that OSA is a very frequent condition among patients with resistant hypertension, and that treatment with CPAP may result in favorable outcomes, that is, reductions in blood pressure, in some patients but not in others.[91–102] The authors found a cluster of plasma miRNAs that can reliably identify the patients who will manifest favorable blood pressure responses to CPAP treatment in the context of resistant hypertension, even if the underlying causes of patient variability in their response to continuous adherent use of CPAP are unknown. Thus, based on the scarce evidence to date, it would seem that the field is prime for studies aimed at identifying differential biomarker plasma or urine-based signatures revolving around the above-mentioned 3 major biomarker-defined target classes.

SINGLE-NUCLEOTIDE POLYMORPHISMS

Single-nucleotide polymorphisms (SNPs) are the most common type of genetic variation among people. Genome-wide association studies build directly on recent efforts to map the patterns of inheritance for the most common form of genomic variation, the SNP.[103,104] Thus far, exploration of risk for developing OSA and susceptibility to OSA-induced morbidities has been the focus of most SNP studies.

For example, OSA is associated with increased risk for metabolic syndrome in both adults and children. In children, the authors found that plasma fatty acid binding protein 4 (FABP4) levels are significantly higher in subjects with OSA when compared with no OSA and after categorizing subjects based on body mass index (BMI) z score.[105] The authors also found not only that increased plasma FABP4 levels correlated with obesity but also that the effect of OSA persists even among obese subjects.[106] In this particular study, the authors explored 11 FABP4 SNPs, which were selected to cover the whole genomic sequence of FABP4, and found that only the rs1054135 polymorphism was significantly more prevalent among OSA as well as among obese children.[106] Taken together, these initial findings in pediatric subjects with OSA suggest that FABP4 SNP (rs1054135) genomic variance may be an important determinant for altered serum FABP4 levels in OSA. Similarly, the macrophage migration inhibitory factor gene (MIF), a pro-inflammatory cytokine that has emerged as a mediator in multiple inflammatory disorders,[107] could be implicated in the morbidity-associated consequences of OSA. Not only was P-OSA associated with higher plasma MIF levels, but also the MIF gene SNP rs10433310 was significantly associated with cardiometabolic risk.[108]

Significant associations between PSG and C-reactive protein (CRP) levels have been identified in children with OSA in several studies, even after adjustment for obesity.[109,110] Furthermore, the link with neurocognitive morbidity and systemic inflammatory responses was further highlighted by the ability to differentiate children with similar OSA severity using plasma CRP levels into those with cognitive deficits and those without.[73] However, there have been several subsequent studies that have failed to replicate these results.[111,112] In order to elucidate the potential source of such discrepant findings, the authors performed a genetic association study that evaluated CRP and interleukin-6 (IL-6) gene variants in P-OSA and found that certain SNP in the CRP and IL-6 genes are related to increased risk for upper airway dysfunction during sleep in the United States, but not in Greece.[74] These latest findings reconciled the reported discrepant CRP levels among the 2 populations as alluded above. The authors hypothesize that the differences in gene variants that significantly associate with OSA between Americans and Greeks might reflect differences in genetic background-environmental exposure interactions leading to divergent disease phenotypes.

To further evaluate genotype-phenotype interactions, the authors examined daytime sleepiness as a robust symptom reporter of underlying susceptibility to OSA. In contrast with A-OSA patients, excessive daytime sleepiness appears not to be as prominent a symptom in children with OSA, with a large proportion of children manifesting "sleepiness" as hyperactive behaviors, impulsivity, and impaired attention and concentration on task. Objective measurements of daytime sleepiness using the Multiple Sleep Latency Test have shown that children with OSA have severity-dependent reductions in sleep latency, but that such reductions in latency are highly variable.[113,114] Furthermore, the magnitude of the reduction in sleep latency is associated with measures of systemic inflammation, such as plasma tumor necrosis factor-α (TNF-α) levels.[115] The results of such studies showed that morning TNF-α levels and Epworth Sleepiness Scale scores are not always increased in the presence of OSA, and that the substantial variability in these measures can be reconciled in the context of polymorphisms in the TNF-α gene that modify the gene transcription.[116] Significant associations were also identified between SNPs of CRP (5237A/G-rs2808630) or glial cell–derived growth factor genes and OSA in European Americans among adult subjects.[117]

OSA is also a risk factor for the occurrence of cardiovascular morbidity. One of the earliest events attesting to such occurrence is the presence of endothelial dysfunction.[118] However, the presence of endothelial dysfunction among children with OSA is highly unpredictable at the individual level.[119] Polymorphisms among genes encoding for nitric oxide synthase and endothelin, which are key regulators of endothelial function, may account for a proportion of such variance in endothelial function.[120,121] In these studies, the authors used genomic DNA from peripheral blood that was extracted from children with and without OSA, and allelic frequencies from custom arrays containing 50,000 SNPs from genetic diversity across approximately 2100 genes related to cardiovascular, inflammatory, hemostasis/coagulation, and metabolic phenotypes and pathways.[121] These

SNPs microarrays contain NOS1 (209 SNPs), NOS2 (122 SNPs), NOS3 (50 SNPs), EDN1 (43 SNPs), EDN2 (48 SNPs), EDN3 (14 SNPs), endothelin receptor A, EDNRA (27 SNPs), and endothelin receptor B, EDNRB (23 SNPs). The relative frequencies of NOS-1, -2, and -3, and EDN-1, -2, -3, -EDNRA, and -EDNRB genotypes were evaluated in 608 subjects (128 with OSA, and 480 without OSA). By comparing no P-OSA vs P-OSA groups, the authors identified 15 differentially distributed SNPs for NOS1 gene and 1 SNP for NOS3, as well as 4 SNPs for EDN1 and 1 SNP for both EDN2 and EDN3.[121] In addition, the authors quantified the mRNA expression of the EDN1 gene in 18 matched subjects, 9 with no P-OSA and 9 with P-OSA using quantitative real-time polymerase chain reaction (qRT-PCR), which confirmed that EDN1 was significantly increased in children with P-OSA (P <.005). These findings suggested that NOS1 and EDN1 genes may confer an increased risk for the presence of P-OSA or downstream morbidity.

Previous research efforts were focused on the identification of gene polymorphisms potentially involved in pathways intermediate to OSA, such as upper airway neuromotor tone, obesity, and inflammation.[122] NADPH (nicotinamide adenine dinucleotide phosphate) oxidase, an enzyme critically involved in free radical formation, has been implicated as a potential cause of neuronal cell loss secondary to intermittent hypoxia during sleep.[123] The authors found that the 242C>T polymorphism in the p22phox subunit of this gene seemingly explains a significant component of the variance in cognitive function phenotype among children with OSA.[124]

In summary, similar to other genomic approaches, the opportunities for identifying gene variants that confer risk for OSA or that enable more precise delineation of morbidity risk deserve further exploration in large-scale cohorts.

EPIGENOMICS

Epigenetics refers to the heritable changes in gene expression without any alterations in DNA sequence. Epigenomics deals with the global analysis of epigenetic changes across the entire genome, in order to reveal the genetic information in addition to the DNA sequence, which may affect gene function. Epigenetic modifications are being increasingly identified as imposing lifelong changes acting at the single- or multiple-gene level and are capable of reprogramming vast areas of the genome if needed. The epigenome is therefore the result of interactions between a given developmental genetic asset and the lifetime actions of the environment.[125] Epigenetic regulation can be implemented by different mechanisms: DNA methylation, histone posttranslational modification, histone variants, RNA interference, and nuclear organization.[57,126–128] Methylation is the most common flexible genomic parameter that can change genome function under exogenous influence and usually occurs in CpG islands, a CG-rich region, in the DNA (eg, promoter regions, regulatory domains, and also intergenic regions).[129] The authors have shown that hypermethylation of CpG dinucleotides in the core promoter region of the eNOS gene was associated with, and likely responsible for, reduced eNOS bioactivity and impaired peripheral vascular function in pediatric patients with OSA.[130]

The authors were also the first to examine DNA methylation in PBMC from children with P-OSA who were matched for gender, ethnicity, BMI, and apnea hypopnea index (AHI), but differed in their plasma levels of CRP.[131] DNA methylation profiling of a panel of 24 major inflammatory-related genes revealed that children with P-OSA and high CRP levels exhibited increased methylation of the FOXP3 gene compared with children with the same P-OSA severity but with normal CRP levels.[131] These findings were confirmed in a larger second-phase case-cohort study that included pyrosequencing of the promoter region of FOXP3. Furthermore, there was a linear correlation between FOXP3 DNA methylation levels and inflammatory markers, such as CRP and myeloid-related protein 8/14 levels, as well as with AHI, as a surrogate reporter of P-OSA severity. Finally, the anticipated hypermethylation of FOXP3 was associated with reduced peripheral counts of T-regulatory cell lymphocytes, the major target of FOXP3 gene transcription.[132,133] Thus, it is likely that epigenetic modifications of selected candidate genes may contribute to the large dispersion of phenotypes in children with OSA.

The concept that epigenetic modifications induced by early life conditions may translate into increased risk for developing OSA is not as farfetched as one might think. Indeed, in a mouse model of late gestation sleep fragmentation mimicking OSA, the authors have shown that offspring of these mothers are at markedly increased risk for developing metabolic syndrome as adults, and that extensive epigenetic changes are present.[134–137] Considering the unique susceptibility of premature infants to develop OSA later in life, epigenetic changes could underlie major components of such risk.[138–140] Thus, specific epigenetic signatures may identify individuals at risk for developing OSA as well as those at risk for manifesting OSA-induced morbidities.

PROTEOMICS

Proteomics is the comprehensive quantitative and functional assessment of all proteins and protein modifications within a certain type of cell, tissue, or body fluid.[141,142] Proteomics complements the research of genome translation and modification and provides a most efficient tool for the comprehensive understanding of gene expression. Two-dimensional gel electrophoresis (2DE) is a traditional early stage approach in proteomics that remains widely used but is less sensitive. The development of high-throughput analytical technologies and quantitative mass spectrometry has enabled a much more precise and extensive exploration of the proteome. In this setting, Shah and colleagues[143] were the first to report that children with OSA may exhibit different protein expression profiles in their serum, and that such differences in proteins or peptides, albeit of unknown identity, provided a diagnostic signature. Plasma levels of malondialdehyde and 8-hydroxy-deoxyguanosine have been shown to be significantly higher in A-OSA patients than in controls, suggesting oxidative stress is greater in OSA patients. Furthermore, levels of these proteins decreased following treatment with CPAP.[144] Subsequent work using iTRAQ proteomic techniques (isobaric tags for relative and absolute quantification) identified a selective number of proteins primarily associated with derangements in lipid and vascular metabolic pathways in A-OSA patients.[145]

Preliminary and encouraging findings in urinary samples obtained from a small sample of children redirected some of the authors' efforts at proteomic biomarker discovery to this easily obtained biological material.[146] In 2 subsequent studies in the authors' laboratory, they examined the urine proteome of P-OSA versus pediatric patients with primary snoring and healthy controls using 2DE.[147] The authors identified 16 unique proteins that were differentially expressed in the OSA group, and ELISA (enzyme-linked immunosorbent assay) validation subsequently confirmed 4 of these proteins (kallikrein-1, urocortin-3, orosomucoid-1, and uromodulin). In a more recent study, the authors developed a proteomics workflow for biomarker discovery based on liquid chromatography–tandem mass spectrometry, an approach that allows for deeper proteome coverage and interrogation of lower-abundance proteins; 192 candidate biomarkers were identified a priori in urine collected from children with P-OSA.[148] Furthermore, using a different protein-based diagnostic panel approach, the authors have recently reported preliminary findings whereby P-OSA manifesting cognitive deficits exhibit different levels of specific neurotransmitters when compared with P-OSA patients without such morbidity.[149] For the sake of completeness, a recent overview of proteomic technologies in the context of OSA was also recently published.[150]

SUMMARY AND FUTURE DIRECTIONS

The quest for biomarkers in OSA is now clearly beyond its initial and tentative launching stages. The costs of diagnosis, the desire to personalize treatment, and the aspirations toward optimized outcomes have all pointed to the need for simpler and more individually tailored processes. In this context, genomics, transcriptomics, and proteomics have led the way, primarily relying on plasma or urine. However, other approaches, such as metabolomics, and alternative samples, such as exhaled breath and saliva, are likely to emerge as viable contenders in the near future. Taken together, the high prevalence of OSA and the seriousness of its consequences completely justify any investments and research efforts targeting the discovery and implementation of biomarker-based clinical algorithms for the diagnosis, risk assessment, and treatment monitoring of OSA patients.

REFERENCES

1. Sehgal A, Mignot E. Genetics of sleep and sleep disorders. Cell 2011;146:194–207.
2. AlGhanim N, Comondore VR, Fleetham J, et al. The economic impact of obstructive sleep apnea. Lung 2008;186:7–12.
3. Mulgrew AT, Ryan CF, Fleetham JA, et al. The impact of obstructive sleep apnea and daytime sleepiness on work limitation. Sleep Med 2007;9:42–53.
4. Swanson LM, Arnedt JT, Rosekind MR, et al. Sleep disorders and work performance: findings from the 2008 National Sleep Foundation Sleep in America poll. J Sleep Res 2011;20:487–94.
5. de Castro JM. The influence of heredity on self-reported sleep patterns in free-living humans. Physiol Behav 2002;76:479–86.
6. Watson NF, Buchwald D, Vitiello MV, et al. A twin study of sleep duration and body mass index. J Clin Sleep Med 2010;6:11–7.
7. Cao C, Ding Q, Lv D, et al. Vascular endothelial growth factor genotypes and haplotypes contribute to the susceptibility of obstructive sleep apnea syndrome. PLoS One 2014;9:e114582.

8. Cao C, Wu B, Wu Y, et al. Functional polymorphisms in the promoter region of MMP-2 and MMP-9 and susceptibility to obstructive sleep apnea. Sci Rep 2015;5:8966.

9. Chi L, Comyn FL, Keenan BT, et al. Heritability of craniofacial structures in normal subjects and patients with sleep apnea. Sleep 2014;37:1689–98.

10. de Lima FF, Mazzotti DR, Tufik S, et al. The role inflammatory response genes in obstructive sleep apnea syndrome: a review. Sleep Breath 2015. [Epub ahead of print].

11. Sun J, Hu J, Tu C, et al. Obstructive sleep apnea susceptibility genes in Chinese population: a field synopsis and meta-analysis of genetic association studies. PLoS One 2015;10:e0135942.

12. Ye R, Yang W, Yuan Y, et al. The CC genotype of the delta-sarcoglycan gene polymorphism rs13170573 is associated with obstructive sleep apnea in the Chinese population. PLoS One 2014;9:e114160.

13. Zhang Y, Li NF, Abulikemu S, et al. Relationship between zinc finger protein 36 (ZFP36) gene polymorphisms and obstructive sleep apnea. Genet Mol Res 2015;14:6733–43.

14. Arnardottir ES, Mackiewicz M, Gislason T, et al. Molecular signatures of obstructive sleep apnea in adults: a review and perspective. Sleep 2009; 32:447–70.

15. Donadio V, Liguori R, Vetrugno R, et al. Daytime sympathetic hyperactivity in OSAS is related to excessive daytime sleepiness. J Sleep Res 2007; 16:327–32.

16. Minoguchi K, Yokoe T, Tazaki T, et al. Increased carotid intima-media thickness and serum inflammatory markers in obstructive sleep apnea. Am J Respir Crit Care Med 2005;172:625–30.

17. Schulz R, Mahmoudi S, Hattar K, et al. Enhanced release of superoxide from polymorphonuclear neutrophils in obstructive sleep apnea. Impact of continuous positive airway pressure therapy. Am J Respir Crit Care Med 2000;162:566–70.

18. Logan AG, Tkacova R, Perlikowski SM, et al. Refractory hypertension and sleep apnoea: effect of CPAP on blood pressure and baroreflex. Eur Respir J 2003;21:241–7.

19. McNicholas WT, Bonsigore MR, Management Committee of EU COST ACTION B26. Sleep apnoea as an independent risk factor for cardiovascular disease: current evidence, basic mechanisms and research priorities. Eur Respir J 2007; 29:156–78.

20. Spruyt K, Gozal D. A mediation model linking body weight, cognition, and sleep-disordered breathing. Am J Respir Crit Care Med 2012;185:199–205.

21. Young T, Palta M, Dempsey J, et al. The occurrence of sleep-disordered breathing among middle-aged adults. N Engl J Med 1993;328: 1230–5.

22. Marcus CL, Brooks LJ, Draper KA, et al, American Academy of Pediatrics. Diagnosis and management of childhood obstructive sleep apnea syndrome. Pediatrics 2012;130:576–84.

23. Lumeng JC, Chervin RD. Epidemiology of pediatric obstructive sleep apnea. Proc Am Thorac Soc 2008;5:242–52.

24. Baldassari CM, Mitchell RB, Schubert C, et al. Pediatric obstructive sleep apnea and quality of life: a meta-analysis. Otolaryngol Head Neck Surg 2008;138:265–73.

25. Bixler EO, Vgontzas AN, Lin HM, et al. Sleep disordered breathing in children in a general population sample: prevalence and risk factors. Sleep 2009; 32:731–6.

26. Crabtree VM, Varni JW, Gozal D. Health-related quality of life and depressive symptoms in children with suspected sleep-disordered breathing. Sleep 2004;27:1131–8.

27. Rosen CL, Larkin EK, Kirchner HL, et al. Prevalence and risk factors for sleep-disordered breathing in 8- to 11-year-old children: association with race and prematurity. J Pediatr 2003;142:383–9.

28. Tauman R, Gozal D. Obesity and obstructive sleep apnea in children. Paediatr Respir Rev 2006;7: 247–59.

29. Gozal D, Pope DW Jr. Snoring during early childhood and academic performance at ages thirteen to fourteen years. Pediatrics 2001;107:1394–9.

30. Capdevila OS, Kheirandish-Gozal L, Dayyat E, et al. Pediatric obstructive sleep apnea: complications, management, and long-term outcomes. Proc Am Thorac Soc 2008;5:274–82.

31. Muzumdar H, Arens R. Physiological effects of obstructive sleep apnea syndrome in childhood. Respir Physiol Neurobiol 2013;188:370–82.

32. Carroll JL, McColley SA, Marcus CL, et al. Inability of clinical history to distinguish primary snoring from obstructive sleep apnea syndrome in children. Chest 1995;108:610–8.

33. Freedman N. COUNTERPOINT: does laboratory polysomnography yield better outcomes than home sleep testing? No. Chest 2015;148:308–10.

34. Kaditis A, Kheirandish-Gozal L, Gozal D. Algorithm for the diagnosis and treatment of pediatric OSA: a proposal of two pediatric sleep centers. Sleep Med 2012;13:217–27.

35. Kaditis A, Kheirandish-Gozal L, Gozal D. Pediatric OSAS: oximetry can provide answers when polysomnography is not available. Sleep Med Rev 2015;27:96–105.

36. Pack AI. POINT: does laboratory polysomnography yield better outcomes than home sleep testing? Yes. Chest 2015;148:306–8.

37. Tan HL, Kheirandish-Gozal L, Gozal D. Pediatric home sleep apnea testing: slowly getting there! Chest 2015;148(6):1382–95.

38. Ralls FM, Grigg-Damberger M. Roles of gender, age, race/ethnicity, and residential socioeconomics in obstructive sleep apnea syndromes. Curr Opin Pulm Med 2012;18:568–73.

39. Yamagishi K, Ohira T, Nakano H, et al. Cross-cultural comparison of the sleep-disordered breathing prevalence among Americans and Japanese. Eur Respir J 2010;36:379–84.

40. Leger D, Bayon V, Laaban JP, et al. Impact of sleep apnea on economics. Sleep Med Rev 2012;16:455–62.

41. Campos-Rodriguez F, Martinez-Garcia MA, Martinez M, et al. Association between obstructive sleep apnea and cancer incidence in a large multicenter Spanish cohort. Am J Respir Crit Care Med 2013;187:99–105.

42. Christensen AS, Clark A, Salo P, et al. Symptoms of sleep disordered breathing and risk of cancer: a prospective cohort study. Sleep 2013;36:1429–35.

43. Nieto FJ, Peppard PE, Young T, et al. Sleep-disordered breathing and cancer mortality: results from the Wisconsin Sleep Cohort Study. Am J Respir Crit Care Med 2012;186:190–4.

44. Kuhle S, Kirk S, Ohinmaa A, et al. Use and cost of health services among overweight and obese Canadian children. Int J Pediatr Obes 2011;6:142–8.

45. Tarasiuk A, Reuveni H. The economic impact of obstructive sleep apnea. Curr Opin Pulm Med 2013;19:639–44.

46. Schwab RJ, Badr SM, Epstein LJ, et al, ATS Subcommittee on CPAP Adherence Tracking Systems. An official American Thoracic Society statement: continuous positive airway pressure adherence tracking systems. The optimal monitoring strategies and outcome measures in adults. Am J Respir Crit Care Med 2013;188:613–20.

47. Weaver TE, Mancini C, Maislin G, et al. Continuous positive airway pressure treatment of sleepy patients with milder obstructive sleep apnea: results of the CPAP Apnea Trial North American Program (CATNAP) randomized clinical trial. Am J Respir Crit Care Med 2012;186:677–83.

48. Lin HS, Zuliani G, Amjad EH, et al. Treatment compliance in patients lost to follow-up after polysomnography. Otolaryngol Head Neck Surg 2007;136:236–40.

49. Simantirakis EN, Schiza SE, Chrysostomakis SI, et al. Atrial overdrive pacing for the obstructive sleep apnea-hypopnea syndrome. N Engl J Med 2005;353:2568–77.

50. Bhattacharjee R, Kheirandish-Gozal L, Spruyt K, et al. Adenotonsillectomy outcomes in treatment of obstructive sleep apnea in children: a multicenter retrospective study. Am J Respir Crit Care Med 2010;182:676–83.

51. Marcus CL, Brooks LJ, Draper KA, et al. Diagnosis and management of childhood obstructive sleep apnea syndrome. Pediatrics 2012;130:e714–55.

52. Kheirandish-Gozal L, Kim J, Goldbart AD, et al. Novel pharmacological approaches for treatment of obstructive sleep apnea in children. Expert Opin Investig Drugs 2013;22:71–85.

53. Gozal D. Serum, urine, and breath-related biomarkers in the diagnosis of obstructive sleep apnea in children: is it for real? Curr Opin Pulm Med 2012;18:561–7.

54. Cavalli-Sforza LL. The human genome diversity project: past, present and future. Nat Rev Genet 2005;6:333–40.

55. Metzker ML. Sequencing technologies—the next generation. Nat Rev Genet 2010;11:31–46.

56. Ozsolak F, Milos PM. RNA sequencing: advances, challenges and opportunities. Nat Rev Genet 2011;12:87–98.

57. Laird PW. Principles and challenges of genome-wide DNA methylation analysis. Nat Rev Genet 2010;11:191–203.

58. Park PJ. ChIP-seq: advantages and challenges of a maturing technology. Nat Rev Genet 2009;10:669–80.

59. Altelaar AF, Munoz J, Heck AJ. Next-generation proteomics: towards an integrative view of proteome dynamics. Nat Rev Genet 2013;14:35–48.

60. Shulaev V. Metabolomics technology and bioinformatics. Brief Bioinformatics 2006;7:128–39.

61. Khalyfa A, Capdevila OS, Buazza MO, et al. Genome-wide gene expression profiling in children with non-obese obstructive sleep apnea. Sleep Med 2009;10:75–86.

62. Hoffmann MS, Singh P, Wolk R, et al. Microarray studies of genomic oxidative stress and cell cycle responses in obstructive sleep apnea. Antioxid Redox Signal 2007;9:661–9.

63. Liew CC, Ma J, Tang HC, et al. The peripheral blood transcriptome dynamically reflects system wide biology: a potential diagnostic tool. J Lab Clin Med 2006;147:126–32.

64. Sullivan PF, Fan C, Perou CM. Evaluating the comparability of gene expression in blood and brain. Am J Med Genet B Neuropsychiatr Genet 2006;141:261–8.

65. Khalyfa A, Gharib SA, Kim J, et al. Peripheral blood leukocyte gene expression patterns and metabolic parameters in habitually snoring and non-snoring children with normal polysomnographic findings. Sleep 2011;34:153–60.

66. Tan HL, Kheirandish-Gozal L, Gozal D. The promise of translational and personalised approaches for paediatric obstructive sleep apnoea: an 'Omics' perspective. Thorax 2014;69:474–80.

67. Gozal D, Serpero LD, Sans Capdevila O, et al. Systemic inflammation in non-obese children with obstructive sleep apnea. Sleep Med 2007;9(3): 254–9.

68. Tauman R, Ivanenko A, O'Brien LM, et al. Plasma C-reactive protein levels among children with sleep-disordered breathing. Pediatrics 2004;113: e564–9.

69. Khalyfa A, Gharib SA, Kim J, et al. Transcriptomic analysis identifies phosphatases as novel targets for adenotonsillar hypertrophy of pediatric obstructive sleep apnea. Am J Respir Crit Care Med 2010; 181:1114–20.

70. Lin SW, Tsai CN, Lee YS, et al. Gene expression profiles in peripheral blood mononuclear cells of Asian obstructive sleep apnea patients. Biomed J 2014;37:60–70.

71. Gharib SA, Hayes AL, Rosen MJ, et al. A pathway-based analysis on the effects of obstructive sleep apnea in modulating visceral fat transcriptome. Sleep 2013;36:23–30.

72. Bjornsdottir E, Janson C, Sigurdsson JF, et al. Symptoms of insomnia among patients with obstructive sleep apnea before and after two years of positive airway pressure treatment. Sleep 2013; 36:1901–9.

73. Gozal D, Crabtree VM, Sans Capdevila O, et al. C-reactive protein, obstructive sleep apnea, and cognitive dysfunction in school-aged children. Am J Respir Crit Care Med 2007;176: 188–93.

74. Kaditis AG, Gozal D, Khalyfa A, et al. Variants in C-reactive protein and IL-6 genes and susceptibility to obstructive sleep apnea in children: a candidate-gene association study in European American and Southeast European populations. Sleep Med 2014;15:228–35.

75. Owens RL, Edwards BA, Eckert DJ, et al. An integrative model of physiological traits can be used to predict obstructive sleep apnea and response to non positive airway pressure therapy. Sleep 2015;38:961–70.

76. Bartel DP. MicroRNAs: genomics, biogenesis, mechanism, and function. Cell 2004;116:281–97.

77. Gilad S, Meiri E, Yogev Y, et al. Serum microRNAs are promising novel biomarkers. PLoS One 2008;3: e3148.

78. Mitchell PS, Parkin RK, Kroh EM, et al. Circulating microRNAs as stable blood-based markers for cancer detection. Proc Natl Acad Sci U S A 2008; 105:10513–8.

79. Krutzfeldt J, Stoffel M. MicroRNAs: a new class of regulatory genes affecting metabolism. Cell Metab 2006;4:9–12.

80. Markham DW, Hill JA. MicroRNAs and heart failure diagnosis: MiR-acle or MiR-age? Circ Res 2010; 106:1011–3.

81. Weber JA, Baxter DH, Zhang S, et al. The microRNA spectrum in 12 body fluids. Clin Chem 2010; 56:1733–41.

82. Zampetaki A, Willeit P, Drozdov I, et al. Profiling of circulating microRNAs: from single biomarkers to re-wired networks. Cardiovasc Res 2012;93:555–62.

83. Zampetaki A, Kiechl S, Drozdov I, et al. Plasma microRNA profiling reveals loss of endothelial miR-126 and other microRNAs in type 2 diabetes. Circ Res 2010;107:810–7.

84. Contu R, Latronico MV, Condorelli G. Circulating microRNAs as potential biomarkers of coronary artery disease: a promise to be fulfilled? Circ Res 2010;107:573–4.

85. Ortega FJ, Mercader JM, Catalan V, et al. Targeting the circulating microRNA signature of obesity. Clin Chem 2013;59:781–92.

86. D'Alessandra Y, Devanna P, Limana F, et al. Circulating microRNAs are new and sensitive biomarkers of myocardial infarction. Eur Heart J 2010;31:2765–73.

87. Khalyfa A, Gozal D. Exosomal miRNAs as potential biomarkers of cardiovascular risk in children. J Transl Med 2014;12:162.

88. Di Stefano V, Zaccagnini G, Capogrossi MC, et al. microRNAs as peripheral blood biomarkers of cardiovascular disease. Vascul Pharmacol 2011; 55:111–8.

89. Khalyfa A, Kheirandish-Gozal L, Bhattacharjee R, et al. Circulating miRNAs as potential biomarkers of endothelial dysfunction in obese children. Chest 2015. [Epub ahead of print].

90. Sanchez-de-la-Torre M, Khalyfa A, Sanchez-de-la-Torre A, et al. Precision medicine in patients with resistant hypertension and obstructive sleep apnea: blood pressure response to continuous positive airway pressure treatment. J Am Coll Cardiol 2015;66:1023–32.

91. Ai J, Epstein PN, Gozal D, et al. Morphology and topography of nucleus ambiguus projections to cardiac ganglia in rats and mice. Neuroscience 2007;149:845–60.

92. Baguet JP, Sosner P, Delsart P, et al. 8c.08: continuous positive airway pressure is efficient to decrease blood pressure in patients with resistant hypertension. Results from the RHOOSAS study. J Hypertens 2015;33(Suppl 1):e112.

93. Barbe F, Duran-Cantolla J, Sanchez-de-la-Torre M, et al. Effect of continuous positive airway pressure on the incidence of hypertension and cardiovascular events in nonsleepy patients with obstructive sleep apnea: a randomized controlled trial. JAMA 2012;307:2161–8.

94. de Abreu-Silva EO, Beltrami-Moreira M. Sleep apnea: an underestimated cause of resistant hypertension. Curr Hypertens Rev 2014;10:2–7.

95. Gunning-Schepers LJ, Hagen JH. Avoidable burden of illness: how much can prevention contribute to health? Soc Sci Med 1987;24:945–51.

96. Iftikhar IH, Valentine CW, Bittencourt LR, et al. Effects of continuous positive airway pressure on blood pressure in patients with resistant hypertension and obstructive sleep apnea: a meta-analysis. J Hypertens 2014;32:2341–50 [discussion: 2350].

97. Martinez-Garcia MA, Capote F, Campos-Rodriguez F, et al, Spanish Sleep Network. Effect of CPAP on blood pressure in patients with obstructive sleep apnea and resistant hypertension: the HIPARCO randomized clinical trial. JAMA 2013; 310:2407–15.

98. Muxfeldt ES, Margallo VS, Guimaraes GM, et al. Prevalence and associated factors of obstructive sleep apnea in patients with resistant hypertension. Am J Hypertens 2014;27:1069–78.

99. Pedrosa RP, Drager LF, de Paula LK, et al. Effects of OSA treatment on BP in patients with resistant hypertension: a randomized trial. Chest 2013;144: 1487–94.

100. Pimenta E, Stowasser M, Gordon RD, et al. Increased dietary sodium is related to severity of obstructive sleep apnea in patients with resistant hypertension and hyperaldosteronism. Chest 2013;143:978–83.

101. Valadi H, Ekstrom K, Bossios A, et al. Exosome-mediated transfer of mRNAs and microRNAs is a novel mechanism of genetic exchange between cells. Nat Cell Biol 2007;9:654–9.

102. Walia HK, Li H, Rueschman M, et al. Association of severe obstructive sleep apnea and elevated blood pressure despite antihypertensive medication use. J Clin Sleep Med 2014;10:835–43.

103. International HapMap Consortium. A haplotype map of the human genome. Nature 2005;437: 1299–320.

104. International HapMap Consortium, Frazer KA, Ballinger DG, Cox DR, et al. A second generation human haplotype map of over 3.1 million SNPs. Nature 2007;449:851–61.

105. Khalyfa A, Bhushan B, Hegazi M, et al. Fatty-acid binding protein 4 gene variants and childhood obesity: potential implications for insulin sensitivity and CRP levels. Lipids Health Dis 2010;9:18.

106. Bhushan B, Khalyfa A, Spruyt K, et al. Fatty-acid binding protein 4 gene polymorphisms and plasma levels in children with obstructive sleep apnea. Sleep Med 2011;12:666–71.

107. Zernecke A, Bernhagen J, Weber C. Macrophage migration inhibitory factor in cardiovascular disease. Circulation 2008;117:1594–602.

108. Khalyfa A, Kheirandish-Gozal L, Capdevila OS, et al. Macrophage migration inhibitory factor gene polymorphisms and plasma levels in children with obstructive sleep apnea. Pediatr Pulmonol 2012; 47:1001–11.

109. Iannuzzi A, Licenziati MR, De Michele F, et al. C-reactive protein and carotid intima-media thickness in children with sleep disordered breathing. J Clin Sleep Med 2013;9:493–8.

110. Ingram DG, Matthews CK. Effect of adenotonsillectomy on C-reactive protein levels in children with obstructive sleep apnea: a meta-analysis. Sleep Med 2013;14:172–6.

111. Kaditis AG, Alexopoulos EI, Kalampouka E, et al. Morning levels of C-reactive protein in children with obstructive sleep-disordered breathing. Am J Respir Crit Care Med 2005;171:282–6.

112. Van Eyck A, Van Hoorenbeeck K, De Winter BY, et al. Sleep-disordered breathing and C-reactive protein in obese children and adolescents. Sleep Breath 2014;18:335–40.

113. Gozal D, Kheirandish-Gozal L. Obesity and excessive daytime sleepiness in prepubertal children with obstructive sleep apnea. Pediatrics 2009; 123:13–8.

114. Gozal D, Wang M, Pope DW Jr. Objective sleepiness measures in pediatric obstructive sleep apnea. Pediatrics 2001;108:693–7.

115. Gozal D, Serpero LD, Kheirandish-Gozal L, et al. Sleep measures and morning plasma TNF-alpha levels in children with sleep-disordered breathing. Sleep 2010;33:319–25.

116. Khalyfa A, Serpero LD, Kheirandish-Gozal L, et al. TNF-alpha gene polymorphisms and excessive daytime sleepiness in pediatric obstructive sleep apnea. J Pediatr 2011;158:77–82.

117. Larkin EK, Patel SR, Goodloe RJ, et al. A candidate gene study of obstructive sleep apnea in European Americans and African Americans. Am J Respir Crit Care Med 2010;182:947–53.

118. Gozal D, Kheirandish-Gozal L, Serpero LD, et al. Obstructive sleep apnea and endothelial function in school-aged nonobese children: effect of adenotonsillectomy. Circulation 2007;116:2307–14.

119. Bhattacharjee R, Kim J, Alotaibi WH, et al. Endothelial dysfunction in children without hypertension: potential contributions of obesity and obstructive sleep apnea. Chest 2012;141: 682–91.

120. Chatsuriyawong S, Gozal D, Kheirandish-Gozal L, et al. Genetic variance in nitric oxide synthase and endothelin genes among children with and without endothelial dysfunction. J Transl Med 2013;11:227.

121. Chatsuriyawong S, Gozal D, Kheirandish-Gozal L, et al. Polymorphisms in nitric oxide synthase and endothelin genes among children with obstructive sleep apnea. BMC Med Genomics 2013;6:29.

122. Riha RL, Brander P, Vennelle M, et al. Tumour necrosis factor-alpha (-308) gene polymorphism

in obstructive sleep apnoea-hypopnoea syndrome. Eur Respir J 2005;26:673–8.

123. Wang Y, Zhang SX, Gozal D. Reactive oxygen species and the brain in sleep apnea. Respir Physiol Neurobiol 2010;174:307–16.

124. Gozal D, Khalyfa A, Capdevila OS, et al. Cognitive function in prepubertal children with obstructive sleep apnea: a modifying role for NADPH oxidase p22 subunit gene polymorphisms? Antioxid Redox Signal 2012;16:171–7.

125. Gluckman PD, Hanson MA, Buklijas T, et al. Epigenetic mechanisms that underpin metabolic and cardiovascular diseases. Nat Rev Endocrinol 2009;5:401–8.

126. Fraser P, Bickmore W. Nuclear organization of the genome and the potential for gene regulation. Nature 2007;447:413–7.

127. Grewal SI, Elgin SC. Transcription and RNA interference in the formation of heterochromatin. Nature 2007;447:399–406.

128. Jenuwein T, Allis CD. Translating the histone code. Science 2001;293:1074–80.

129. Sandoval J, Esteller M. Cancer epigenomics: beyond genomics. Curr Opin Genet Dev 2012; 22:50–5.

130. Kheirandish-Gozal L, Khalyfa A, Gozal D, et al. Endothelial dysfunction in children with obstructive sleep apnea is associated with epigenetic changes in the eNOS gene. Chest 2013;143:971–7.

131. Kim J, Bhattacharjee R, Khalyfa A, et al. DNA methylation in inflammatory genes among children with obstructive sleep apnea. Am J Respir Crit Care Med 2012;185:330–8.

132. Tan HL, Gozal D, Samiei A, et al. T regulatory lymphocytes and endothelial function in pediatric obstructive sleep apnea. PLoS One 2013;8: e69710.

133. Tan HL, Gozal D, Wang Y, et al. Alterations in circulating T-cell lymphocyte populations in children with obstructive sleep apnea. Sleep 2013;36:913–22.

134. Cortese R, Khalyfa A, Bao R, et al. Epigenomic profiling in visceral white adipose tissue of offspring of mice exposed to late gestational sleep fragmentation. Int J Obes 2015;39:1135–42.

135. Khalyfa A, Carreras A, Almendros I, et al. Sex dimorphism in late gestational sleep fragmentation and metabolic dysfunction in offspring mice. Sleep 2015;38:545–57.

136. Khalyfa A, Mutskov V, Carreras A, et al. Sleep fragmentation during late gestation induces metabolic perturbations and epigenetic changes in adiponectin gene expression in male adult offspring mice. Diabetes 2014;63:3230–41.

137. Mutskov V, Khalyfa A, Wang Y, et al. Early-life physical activity reverses metabolic and Foxo1 epigenetic misregulation induced by gestational sleep disturbance. Am J Physiol Regul Integr Comp Physiol 2015;308:R419–30.

138. Huang YS, Guilleminault C. Pediatric obstructive sleep apnea and the critical role of oral-facial growth: evidences. Front Neurol 2012;3:184.

139. Poets CF, Khan SR. Former preterm infants, caffeine was good for you, but now beware of snoring! Am J Respir Crit Care Med 2014;190:720–1.

140. Sharma PB, Baroody F, Gozal D, et al. Obstructive sleep apnea in the formerly preterm infant: an overlooked diagnosis. Front Neurol 2011;2:73.

141. Anderson NL, Anderson NG. Proteome and proteomics: new technologies, new concepts, and new words. Electrophoresis 1998;19:1853–61.

142. Blackstock WP, Weir MP. Proteomics: quantitative and physical mapping of cellular proteins. Trends Biotechnol 1999;17:121–7.

143. Shah ZA, Jortani SA, Tauman R, et al. Serum proteomic patterns associated with sleep-disordered breathing in children. Pediatr Res 2006;59:466–70.

144. Jurado-Gamez B, Fernandez-Marin MC, Gomez-Chaparro JL, et al. Relationship of oxidative stress and endothelial dysfunction in sleep apnoea. Eur Respir J 2011;37:873–9.

145. Jurado-Gamez B, Gomez-Chaparro JL, Munoz-Calero M, et al. Serum proteomic changes in adults with obstructive sleep apnoea. J Sleep Res 2012;21:139–46.

146. Krishna J, Shah ZA, Merchant M, et al. Urinary protein expression patterns in children with sleep-disordered breathing: preliminary findings. Sleep Med 2006;7:221–7.

147. Gozal D, Jortani S, Snow AB, et al. Two-dimensional differential in-gel electrophoresis proteomic approaches reveal urine candidate biomarkers in pediatric obstructive sleep apnea. Am J Respir Crit Care Med 2009;180:1253–61.

148. Becker L, Kheirandish-Gozal L, Peris E, et al. Contextualised urinary biomarker analysis facilitates diagnosis of paediatric obstructive sleep apnoea. Sleep Med 2014;15:541–9.

149. Kheirandish-Gozal L, McManus CJ, Kellermann GH, et al. Urinary neurotransmitters are selectively altered in children with obstructive sleep apnea and predict cognitive morbidity. Chest 2013;143: 1576–83.

150. Feliciano A, Torres VM, Vaz F, et al. Overview of proteomics studies in obstructive sleep apnea. Sleep Med 2015;16:437–45.

Novel Therapies for the Treatment of Central Sleep Apnea

Shahrokh Javaheri, MD[a],*, Robin Germany, MD[b],
John J. Greer, PhD[c]

KEYWORDS

- Congestive heart failure • Opioids • Ampakines • CPAP • Adaptive servo ventilators • Apnea

KEY POINTS

- Central sleep apnea (CSA), rare in general population, is a common polysomographic finding in patients with heart failure and chronic opioid users.
- Adaptive servoventilation devices have been successfully used to treat central sleep apnea in both heart failure and with opioids.
- A recent study using an out dated adaptive servoventilation failed to show benefits in treating CSA in heart failure.

INTRODUCTION

Neurophysiologically, central sleep apnea (CSA) is due to a temporary failure of respiratory rhythmogenesis. CSA occurs in a number of disorders across all age groups and both genders.[1] The most common causes of CSA are cardiocerebrovascular disorders, such as congestive heart failure, atrial fibrillation, and stroke, and chronic use of opioids to treat pain. In this article, the authors concentrate on the treatment of CSA in heart failure (HF) and in association with opioids. There have been important advances in the therapy of CSA in these 2 conditions.

At the outset, it is emphasized that the patterns of breathing associated with CSA due to HF versus opioids are distinctly different from each other, as shown in **Figs. 1** and **2** and later discussed. This distinction is diagnostically important because the therapeutic options are distinctly different for these 2 conditions.

CENTRAL SLEEP APNEA AND PERIODIC BREATHING IN HEART FAILURE

CSA in HF, with both reduced and preserved ejection fraction (HFrEF and HFpEF, respectively), occurs in the background of a unique periodic breathing referred to as Hunter-Cheyne-Stokes breathing (HCSB)[2] (see **Fig. 1**). The pattern was first recognized by John Hunter several decades before John Cheyne noted it (see Ref.[2] for details). This crescendo-decrescendo pattern of breathing occurs primarily in non-rapid eye movement (REM) sleep and is related to increased loop gain, which is present in a subset of patients with HF.[1,3,4] Central apneas and hypopneas frequently occur between the crescendo-decrescendo arms of periodic breathing. These events are associated with arterial oxyhemoglobin desaturation, changes in partial pressure of carbon dioxide, and arousals. These pathophysiological consequences of HCSB eventually result in a hyperadrenergic state, which is a

[a] Bethesda North Hospital, 10535 Montgomery Road, Suite 200, Cincinnati, OH 45242, USA; [b] Section of Cardiology, University of Oklahoma College of Medicine, Oklahoma City, OK, USA; [c] University of Alberta, Edmonton, Alberta, Canada
* Corresponding author.
E-mail address: shahrokhjavaheri@icloud.com

Sleep Med Clin 11 (2016) 227–239
http://dx.doi.org/10.1016/j.jsmc.2016.01.004
1556-407X/16/$ – see front matter © 2016 Elsevier Inc. All rights reserved.

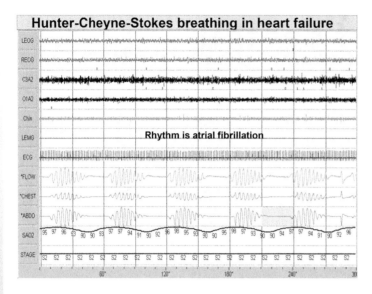

Fig. 1. A 5-minute epoch of a polysomnogram of a patient with systolic HF showing HCSB with central apneas in N2 non-REM sleep. Note the gradual decrease in ABD and chest tracings followed by a gradual symmetric increase in these tracings out of central apnea sandwiched between the thoracoabdominal excursions. ABDO, abdomen; ECG, electrocardiogram; EEG, electroencephalogram; EOG, electro-oculogram; thermocouple tracing representing airflow, SaO_2, arterial oxyhemoglobin saturation. (*Adapted from* Javaheri S. Heart failure. In: Kryger MH, Roth T, Dement WC, editors. Principles and practices of sleep medicine. 6th edition. Philadelphia: WB Saunders, in press; with permission.)

known predictor of premature mortality in patients with HF. HF patients with CSA have excess hospital readmission,[5] and mortality, when compared with HF patients without CSA.[6] Therefore, the hope has been that treatment of CSA in HF would attenuate the number of hospital readmissions and premature mortality. However, as will be noted later, a recent phase 3 randomized clinical trial using the old generation adaptive servoventilation (ASV), to treat CSA in HFrEF failed to show any improvement in either hospitalization or all-cause mortality.

PREVALENCE OF CENTRAL SLEEP APNEA IN HEART FAILURE

There are many studies from different laboratories and from many countries that have consistently shown high prevalence of CSA in patients with HF with both reduced and preserved in left ventricular ejection fraction (LVEF) (for reviews see Refs.[1,2]). In these studies, the prevalence of predominant CSA as a disorder varies from 20% to 50% of the consecutive patients enrolled. These

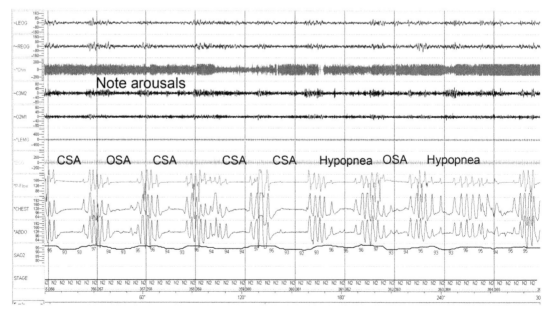

Fig. 2. A typical 5-minute epoch of various disordered breathing events associated with the use of opioids. Note central apneas of variable duration (contrast **Fig. 1**), large breaths out of apnea (contrast **Fig. 1**). Tracings similar to **Fig. 1**. (*Adapted from* Javaheri S, Malik A, Smith J, et al. Adaptive pressure support servoventilation: a novel treatment for sleep apnea associated with use of opioids. J Clin Sleep Med 2008;4(4):305–10; with permission.)

patients had an apnea hypopnea index (AHI) of 15 or more per hour of sleep. The reasons for this huge variation are multiple, including classification of hypopneas as obstructive or central. Obstructive or central is important, because commonly, most of the sleep-disordered breathing events are hypopneas. Sleep apnea is underdiagnosed in patients with HF.[7] In this cohort of Medicare beneficiaries, only 2% of about 30,000 patients with HF were tested for sleep apnea. Those who were tested were diagnosed and treated for sleep apnea and had improved survival and less hospitalization.

A similar prevalence of sleep-disordered breathing has been reported in patients with HF and HFpEF.[8,9] In the largest study,[8] 244 consecutive patients (87 women) with well-documented HFpEF underwent cardiac catheterization and polygraphy. Forty-eight percent of the patients had an AHI of 15 or more per hour of recording, of whom 25% had obstructive sleep apnea (OSA) and 23% had CSA. Therefore, the prevalence of CSA remains high when consecutive patients with HF, irrespective of presence or absence of symptoms undergo a sleep study.

A higher prevalence of sleep-related breathing disorders has been reported in patients with acute decompensated HF. Khayat and coworkers[10] performed a prospective cohort study of patients hospitalized with acute heart failure (AHF) in a single academic heart hospital. During a 4-year period, from 2007 to 2010, all patients hospitalized with AHF who had LVEF ≤ 45% and were not already diagnosed with sleep apnea underwent cardiopulmonary sleep testing while in the hospital (second or third night). One thousand one hundred eleven hospitalized AHF patients had successful sleep testing. Using an AHI of 15 or more per hour of recording, 78% of the patients had moderate to severe sleep apnea, 47% with OSA and 31% with CSA.

TREATMENT OF CENTRAL SLEEP APNEA IN HEART FAILURE

The treatment options for CSA are evolving (for reviews, see Refs.[2,11,12]). In general, however, CSA is more difficult to treat than OSA. Not surprisingly therefore, various positive airway pressure (PAP) devices, including continuous positive airway pressure (CPAP), bilevel, and ASV devices, and multiple medications have been tried. With virtually all of these therapeutic options, significant residual events may remain.

To begin with, optimization of cardiopulmonary function, both pharmacologic, diuretics, angiotensin converting enzyme inhibitors, and β-blockers, and nonpharmacologic cardiac resynchronization therapy, have been shown to improve CSA. However, HF is a progressive disease, and with progression, CSA may emerge or worsen.

The best therapeutic option is cardiac transplantation, as reported elsewhere.[13] However, many cardiac transplant recipients develop OSA due to weight gain, and those who gain the most are most prone to develop OSA.[13] In the authors' study, cardiac transplant patients with OSA also developed hypertension and had poor quality of life compared with those without OSA.[13]

Among the various potential options to treat CSA in HF, 2 specific devices (PAP devices including the CPAP device and adaptive Servo ventilation), and a transvenous pacemaker device, that stimulates the phrenic nerve while the patient is asleep, preventing the occurrence of central apneas, are discussed.[14]

POSITIVE AIRWAY PRESSURE IN THE TREATMENT OF CENTRAL SLEEP APNEA IN HEART FAILURE

Noninvasive PAP devices, including CPAP, bilevel, and ASV, have been used in multiple studies to treat predominant CSA in patients with HF.[2,12,13] In the only long-term multicenter Canadian trial, CPAP therapy did not improve overall survival of HFrEF patients with CSA.[15] The trial was prematurely terminated for several reasons, including reduced mortality due to introduction of β-blockers in the medical treatment of HF, and most importantly, because of early divergence of the survival curves in favor of the control group ($P = .02$), even though the overall survival was not significant. In this study, the main reasons for mortality were pump failure and sudden death, the 2 most common modes of demise in HF. In their initial analysis,[15] the investigators did not categorize HF patients into CPAP responders versus nonresponders. In a pro-and-con discussion[16] and based on previous observations,[17] the authors suggested that excess mortality was primarily in nonresponders. A later post-hoc analysis[18] of the data showed significant improvement in survival of CPAP responders. The reasons for CPAP-induced increased mortality are multiple, including adverse hemodynamic effects of increased intrathoracic pressure (decreasing venous return and cardiac output), which in patients who continue to have persistent CSA on CPAP could be deleterious. It must be emphasized, however, that attenuation of CSA in the group of the CPAP responders could also have been in part due to improved cardiac function with the use of CPAP, and, as noted above, the addition of β-blockers to the armamentarium of pharmacotherapy of HF during the trial. Regarding the former, CPAP by itself, in the absence of CSA or without improving CSA, does not improve cardiac function as measured by LVEF and does not affect survival. However, β-blockers do improve cardiac function. Therefore, a better analysis of survival would have been between CPAP responders versus individuals in the control group in whom cardiac function improved with the addition of β-blockers. A later study[19] showed that only 18 of the 98 patients showed improved cardiac function when β-blockers were added. Despite the small number, it is of interest to see if CSA improved in these patients. Another concern is that initially there were 130 patients on CPAP, and the post-hoc analysis included only 100 patients.

ASV devices are the most advanced of PAP devices.[20] They interfere most precisely with the pathophysiology of HCSB. The algorithms apply variable inspiratory pressure support (defined as the pressure difference between inspiratory and expiratory pressures) according to the actual requirements of the patient throughout the night. The inspiratory pressure support is increased during periods of hypoventilation and reduced during hyperventilation. It is emphasized however that the algorithm of inspiratory pressure support is engaged when the patient's ventilation decreases to less than 90% to 95% of the most recent patient's ventilation. At the same time, it is noted that the algorithm of the older generation of ASV devices dictated an obligatory minimum inspiratory pressure support of 3 cm of water above the prevailing end-expiratory pressure, no matter the level of the end-expiratory pressure. This device was used in the ResMed SERVE-HF trial to be discussed later. Another feature of all ASV devices is delivery of mandatory breaths applied to avoid central apneas in the face of a lack of timely spontaneous inspiration. The most advanced algorithms also apply variable expiratory pressure to adapt to changing levels of upper airway obstruction. This automatic variable pressure is in contrast to CPAP devices and should provide most comfort for the patients.

Multiple studies have consistently proven the efficacy of ASV devices to suppress CSA/HCSB,[12,21–23] and observational studies show improved survival of HF patients who use the device compared with those who refused or were intolerant. These devices are also effective in coexisting obstructive and central disturbances in cardiac patients. As a result of positive outcomes of these observational studies, 2 large,

randomized clinical trials with ASV were designed. In one of these trials, which is ongoing (ADVENT-HF, Effect of ASV on Survival and Hospital Admissions in HF, NCT01128816), HF patients with either OSA or CSA are being enrolled. In the ADVENT-HF trial, a Philips Respironics ASV device (Murrysville, PA, USA) is used, and this device is equipped with auto expiratory PAP capable of treating both OSA and CSA. Furthermore, as detailed elsewhere,[20] the algorithms of this device are different from that of ResMed ASV devices. Importantly, so far, there has been no signal of excess mortality in the ASV arm of the ADVENT-HF trial. The second already completed trial enrolled HF patients with predominantly CSA (SERVE-HF, Treatment of Predominant CSA by ASV in Patients with HF, NCT00733343). The SERVE-HF[24] is a multicenter randomized controlled trial designed to compare the effect of standard medical management plus ASV versus medical management alone in patients with symptomatic chronic HF with HFrEF, LVEF ≤45%, and mostly class III patients (some class IV, and class II with at least one hospitalization for HF over the preceding 24 months were also enrolled). Patients underwent polygraphy or polysomnography. Patients enrolled had an AHI ≥15 events per hour of recording, in the case of both polygraphy and polysomnography. Predominant CSA was defined as more than 50% central events and central AHI ≥10. The primary endpoint was all-cause mortality or unplanned hospitalization for HF. A total of 1325 patients were randomized and followed for a mean of 3.5 years. The study cost was approximately US$38 million. The preliminary results were made public on May 13, 2015, and the article was published recently.[24] There was no statistically significant difference in the primary endpoint (hazard ratio [HR] = 1.14, 95% confidence interval [CI]: 0.97–1.33, $P = .10$). With the hope of finding a positive secondary outcome, unfortunately the investigators discovered a statistically significant increased risk of cardiovascular mortality with ASV compared with control: there was a 2.5% absolute increase in the annual cardiovascular mortality associated with use of ASV compared with medical therapy alone (10% per year in ASV compared with 7.5% per year in controls, HR = 1.34, 95% CI: 1.07–1.67, $P = .01$). Therefore, not only was ASV ineffective, but also its use was actually associated with excess cardiovascular mortality. ResMed advised clinicians that use of ASV is contraindicated for treatment of predominantly CSA in patients with symptomatic HF and reduced LVEF. It must be emphasized that this excess mortality was independent of whether the patients felt improved or not. The authors have been told that most patients died during daytime and some during sleep. The breakdown of these patients remains to be published, and there may have been different reasons for nocturnal versus diurnal deaths. Following the ResMed (San Diego, CA, USA) report, Philips Respironics, the maker of a different ASV device, also declared a contraindication for the use of their device in patients with the phenotype similar to those in the SERVE-HF trial.

Therefore, in the 2 randomized clinical trials, one with CPAP and the other with an ASV, there is excess mortality associated with the use of the PAP device. The history repeats itself. However, it should be emphasized that at least on the surface, the reasons for mortality and also the mode of mortality are different in the 2 trials. First, regarding mortality, in the Canadian CPAP trial, the excess mortality associated with CPAP was in the subset in which CSA was not suppressed by CPAP. In contrast, patients in whom CSA was suppressed by CPAP had better survival than the control group. In the SERVE-HF trial, the investigators have reported that AHI significantly improved. However, ASV is not uniformly effective,[25] and it is conceivable that this subset of patients contributed, in part, to excess mortality. In that case, the scenario is similar to that of the Canadian trial with CPAP. In the Canadian trial, in patients using CPAP and in whom survival improved, cardiovascular function also improved. In contrast, in those patients in whom use of CPAP was associated with excess mortality, cardiovascular function did not improve. Therefore, the question arises if in the SEVE-HF trial, there are 2 subsets of patients in the ASV arm, one subgroup with improved cardiac function, and the other subset in whom use of ASV was not associated with improved, or perhaps worsening of, cardiac function. A post-hoc analysis of these subgroups could shed light on this question. In this regard, it is conceivable that in some patients with HF in whom right ventricular stroke volume is preload dependent, increased intrathoracic pressure with the use of an ASV device could result in worsening cardiac function as suggested in the case of the Canadian trial.[16] Specifically, in patients with HF who develop combined postcapillary and precapillary pulmonary hypertension, right ventricular systolic dysfunction emerges. It is this subset of HF patients who are particularly vulnerable to increased intrathoracic pressure when PAP is applied. It should be further emphasized that increased intrathoracic pressure may also increase pulmonary vascular resistance by increasing the lung volume with a consequent

increase in pulmonary vascular resistance. A combination of decreasing preload and increasing afterload of the right ventricle with the use of ASV, again in some patients with HF, could also contribute to excess mortality. In this regard, in SERVE-HF, the old generation ResMed ASV (which is no longer manufactured in the United States) was used, and in this device, a mandatory minimum inspiratory pressure support is continuously (during inspiration) applied. In contrast, in the new generation ResMed ASV device, and in the Philips Respironics ASV device, minimum pressure support could be set at 0. This setting may be important because periodic breathing in HF is virtually absent in REM sleep, and pressure support is not necessary and may be hazardous. There are other potential factors that might have contributed to the negative results of the SERVR-HF trial.[24] Meanwhile, as more is learned of the details of the SERVE-HF, potentially other reasons explaining the increased mortality in the ASV arm may become evident.

TRANSVENOUS PHRENIC NERVE STIMULATION FOR TREATMENT OF CENTRAL SLEEP APNEA IN HEART FAILURE

A new approach to the treatment of CSA, designed to address the underlying pathophysiology of the disease (lack of signaling from the brain to breathe when appropriate), has been developed.[14] This new device (the remedē System; Respicardia, Inc, Minnetonka, MN, USA; **Fig. 3**) uses a neurostimulation approach to stimulate the phrenic nerve and move the diaphragm.[14] The stimulation algorithm is designed to restore normal breathing, oxygenation, and sleep in

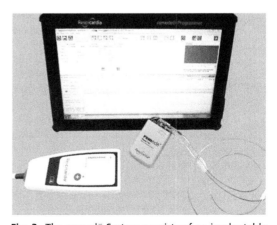

Fig. 3. The remedē System consists of an implantable neurostimulator, stimulation lead, programmer and programming wand. (*Courtesy of* Respicardia, Inc, Minnetonka, MN; with permission.)

patients with CSA by stabilization of oxygen and CO_2 levels and prevent cyclical breathing.[14,24,26] By using the normal stimulation pathway, changes in pressure and volume are similar to those seen in normal breathing. The fully implantable remedē System includes a stimulation lead and an implanted neurostimulator and is implanted in a similar manner to a cardiac pacemaker (**Fig. 4**). The stimulation lead is implanted in either the left pericardiophrenic or the right brachiocephalic vein with unique lead configurations for each location. The neurostimulator is placed subcutaneously under the collarbone in either the left or the right pectoral region to allow for concomitant cardiac device implantation.[24]

Once implanted, the System is programmed and monitored via a tablet-type programmer. Individualized settings, including start and stop times, and maximum stimulation are programmed based on patient feedback and overnight monitoring. Once programmed, the remedē System automatically activates each night.

Initial data with the remedē System demonstrated that the concept improved CSA acutely. An early study showed improvement in AHI, oxygen, and carbon dioxide with acute therapy.[26] Following this initial study, a larger feasibility study was started. Patients underwent temporary stimulation lead placement and were monitored for 2 nights. For each patient, a stimulation night was compared with a control night. Evaluation

revealed a 50% improvement AHI as well as improvements in oxygen and arousals.[14] The study also confirmed that stimulation was well tolerated by patients and led to the development of the fully implantable system, which was tested in a small safety study.[27]

A multinational chronic pilot study was completed using the fully implantable system.[28] The patient population was older (65.9 ± 9.6 years) with low body mass index (29.3 ± 4.4 kg/m^2) and ejection fraction ($30.5 \pm 11.6\%$). Similar to other studies in CSA, patients were predominantly men (89%). Many patients had significant comorbidities, including HF (79%), atrial fibrillation (30%), and hypertension (74%). In addition, 50% of patients had a concomitant implanted cardiac rhythm device. The study showed an 82% reduction in central apnea events (29 ± 14 to 5 ± 9 events per hour) and a 56% reduction in AHI (from 50 ± 15 to 22 ± 14 events per hour) at 3 months (**Fig. 5**). In addition, significant reductions in oxygen desaturation (50%) and arousals (31%) were noted. Patients also had symptomatic benefit as demonstrated by improvement in the patient global assessment scale, Epworth Sleepiness Scale, and the Minnesota Living with Heart Failure Scale (in patients with HF). Improvements were maintained through 6 months. There were several patients early in the study with a need for lead repositioning or difficulty with lead placement, but this improved over the course of the study with improved implantation

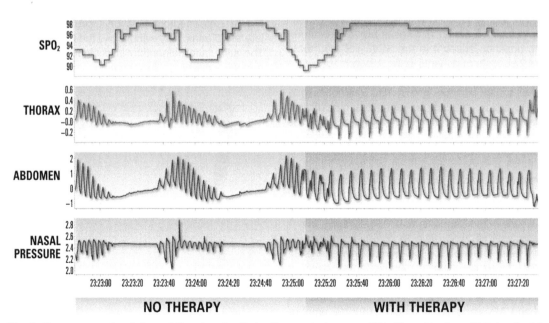

Fig. 4. Transvenous stimulation of the phrenic eliminating central apneas CSA. (*From* Ponikowski P, Javaheri S, Michalkiewicz D, et al. Transvenous phrenic nerve stimulation for the treatment of central sleep apnea in heart failure. Eur Heart J 2012;33:889–94.)

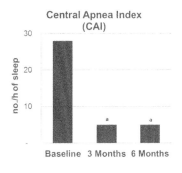

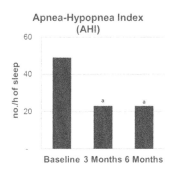

Fig. 5. Effects of transvenous phrenic nerve stimulation at 3 and 6 months. [a] All changes are statistically significant at 3 and 6 months by paired Student t test ($P<.0001$). N = 44. (Data from Abraham WT, Jagielski D, Oldenburg O, et al. Phrenic nerve stimulation for the treatment of central sleep apnea. JACC Heart Fail 2015;5:360–6.)

techniques. This experience was similar to other newly developed transvenous stimulation devices. The investigators concluded that the benefit of this therapeutic approach outweighed the risk of implantation of the device and recommended that a randomized controlled trial be conducted.[14]

Currently, a worldwide, randomized controlled pivotal trial is ongoing (NCT01816776) and will compare patients receiving the remedē System therapy with an implanted control group without therapy at 6 months. Safety will be evaluated through 12 months. A variety of secondary endpoints will be examined, including sleep metrics, cardiovascular markers (echocardiography and heart rate variability), as well as quality of life.[29]

The remedē System offers a unique approach to treating CSA by targeting the disrupted breathing pathway in the body and working to restore this pathway. By using this approach, the therapeutic effect on other systems, such as that seen with medications, should be minimized. In addition, by preventing the hypoxia and arousals associated with CSA, it is anticipated that improvements in comorbidities will continue to be demonstrated long term.

OPIOIDS-INDUCED CENTRAL SLEEP APNEA

In recent years, use of opioid medications has increased dramatically in part due to an increased awareness by health care providers to treat chronic pain, and patients' awareness to seek treatment. From 1990 to 1996, the use of opioids has increased for 4 opioid analgesics: fentanyl, morphine, oxycodone, and hydromorphone by 1168%, 59%, 23%, and 19%, respectively.[30] Similarly, from 1997 to 2003, therapeutic use of methadone and oxycodone has increased by 824% and 660%, respectively.[31] In addition to increased therapeutic use, an estimated 4.7 million individuals are using opioids illegally.[32] Meanwhile, use of opioids has been associated with increased mortality.[33] The spectrum of sleep-related breathing disorders due to opioids is considered an important cause of mortality

because patients are found dead in bed, and no cause is found postmortem.[34]

Opioid-induced CSA occurs in 2 specific circumstances. First, CSA may be found during initial polysomnographic study, which proves to be CPAP resistant, and second, CSA may emerge with CPAP therapy in individuals with OSA. The latter is referred to as complex sleep apnea. These 2 phenotypes of CSA are discussed as follows:

A. CSA presents during initial polysomnographic study. These patients may present with symptoms suggestive of OSA, but polysomnography shows the presence of either CSA as the predominant form of sleep apnea or CSA mixed with both obstructive sleep apneas and hypopneas.[35–40] The pattern of breathing and CSA associated with chronic opioid use has unique characteristics.[35,36] Data from studies using polysomnograms suggest that opioid-induced sleep-disordered breathing is characterized by several respiratory patterns. The more common pattern seen in opioid-induced CSA is cluster breathing, characterized by cycles of deep breaths in which the amplitude of tidal volume is relatively stable with interspersed central apneas of variable duration (see Fig. 2). Another pattern is ataxic breathing characterized by variable amplitude in tidal volume and breathing rate. Similar to the observation in HF, with opioids, CSA occurs primarily in non-REM sleep. The prevalence of CSA, defined as a central apnea index (CAI) $\geq$ 5 per hour of sleep, is estimated to vary from 11% to 36% in patients on chronic opioids (see Refs.[41–43] for review). In contrast, it is estimated that in the general population invariably CAI is less than 1 per hour of sleep.

B. Opioids are associated with the complex sleep apnea. In this condition, central apneas emerge during initiation of CPAP therapy. Specifically, CSA was not present during initial diagnostic polysomnography. These individuals present with the symptoms and signs associated with OSA, which is confirmed by polysomnography, and central apneas emerge and remain persistent with continued use of CPAP.[44] The authors first noticed this in a large series of patients who presented with OSA without or with a few central apneas during initial polysomnography. However, central apneas (CAI $\geq$ 5) emerged on commencement of CPAP therapy and persisted despite continued use of CPAP; this occurred mostly in patients on opioids. In most of the remaining patients with OSA, except for a few, CSA disappeared with continued use of CPAP. This finding was confirmed in a case control study of patients on chronic opioids, with polysomnographic evidence of severe OSA (mean AHI 44/h, mean CAI = 0.6 ± 1.4/h of sleep)[45] and with the emergence of a high rate of central apneas (mean CAI = 14/h) with CPAP treatment.

TREATMENT OPTIONS FOR OPIOID-INDUCED CENTRAL SLEEP APNEA

From practical and theoretic considerations, there are several options. When possible, supervised withdrawal of opioids should eliminate CSA, but this is difficult to achieve.

Two therapeutic options, PAP devices and the pharmacologic approach of ampakine administration, are discussed.

Positive Airway Pressure Devices

Multiple studies,[36,40,44–46] with one exception,[47] have shown disappointing results when CPAP was applied for the treatment of CSA in chronic opioid users, this despite continued use of CPAP.[36] The authors have discontinued using CPAP for treatment of opioids-induced CSA. Better results have been obtained with bilevel with backup rate or ASV devices.[25,36,48] Volume-assured ventilation should be effective as well, but the authors are not aware of any systematic studies.

ASV devices have been studied the most thoroughly. Allam and coworkers[45] performed a retrospective study of 100 patients who failed conventional CPAP therapy for various types of CSA, including those due to opioids. These patients were successfully treated with an ASV device.

Javaheri and coworkers[36] reported 20 patients who presented with symptoms of OSA, but on full-night attended polysomnography proved to have severe hybrid sleep apnea with a large number of CSA being present (AHI = 70, CAI = 26). Most of these patients had persistent CSA on commencement of CPAP therapy, and CSA index

remained unchanged in 9 of the 20 patients who continued to use CPAP for several weeks. These patients remained symptomatic. This reason was, as noted earlier, that the authors stopped recommending CPAP for opioids-induced CSA. All patients were effectively treated with ASV and continued to be adherent over the long term.[36] ASV may be superior to bilevel with a backup rate. In a prospective, randomized crossover study, Cao and colleagues[46] studied 18 consecutive patients (age $\geq$ 18 years) who had been receiving opioid therapy ($\geq$6 months) and had sleep-disordered breathing with CSA (CAI $\geq$ 5) diagnosed during an overnight polysomnography or PAP titration. They were enrolled to undergo 2 polysomnography studies—one with ASVAuto and one with bilevel-ST. Patients suffered from severe sleep apnea (AHI = 50 and CAI = 13). Comparing the 2 devices, sleep-related disordered breathing events were significantly lower with ASVAuto than with bilevel-ST (AHI 2.5 vs 16, $P = .0005$, and CAI, 0.4 vs 9, $P = .0002$). Patients felt more awake and alert on ASVAuto than bilevel-ST based on scores from the Morning After Patient Satisfaction Questionnaire ($P = .03$).

It must be emphasized that ASV is not uniformly effective. In the above study, ASV resolved sleep-disordered breathing in 83% of the patients. In an earlier study, Ramar and colleagues[25] reported that ASV was successful in 28 (60%) of the 47 patients on opioids These patients had severe sleep apnea with an AHI of 48 and CAI of 18 per hour of sleep. In this study, success was defined if AHI decreased less than 10 per hour of sleep.

Regarding complex sleep apnea, Guilleminault and coworkers[48] performed a case control study in 44 chronic opioid users with severe OSA (mean AHI = 44, CAI = 0.6/h of sleep). The investigators observed a high rate of central apneas on treatment with CPAP (CAI = 14/h) and bilevel (CAI = 12/h). However, bilevel with backup respiratory rate (bilevel ST) effectively eliminated central apneas (CAI = 2/h) and obstructive apneas, improved nocturnal oxyhemoglobin saturation and daytime sleepiness.

AMPAKINE THERAPY FOR COUNTERING CENTRAL RESPIRATORY DEPRESSION

There is an emerging body of data demonstrating that a class of drugs called ampakines can alleviate respiratory depression related to drugs, disease, and weak endogenous drive.[49–55] The efficacy against opioid-induced respiratory depression has been best characterized and includes both rodent and human studies.[49,50,55] The basics of respiratory control that provided the foundation for the hypothesis that ampakines would stimulate weak respiratory drive, an overview of ampakines, and preclinical and clinical data related to ampakines and respiratory depression are discussed, with an emphasis on opioids.

Respiratory Neural Control and the Importance of Amino-3-hydroxy-5-methyl-4-isoxazolepropionate Receptor Activation

The neurotransmitter glutamate is critical for the generation of respiratory rhythm within the pre-BotC.[56–59] Ionotropic glutamate receptors are separated into 3 functionally distinct subclasses: Amino-3-hydroxy-5-methyl-4-isoxazolepropionate (AMPA), kainite, and NMDA (N-methyl-D-aspartate). Activation of all 3 of these glutamate receptor subtypes will modulate respiratory rhythmogenesis, but it is activation via AMPA receptors that is a key regulator of pre-BötC function. The inspiratory rhythmogenic drive generated by the preBötC is transmitted via a series of synaptic connections to cranial and spinal motoneurons that in turn activate respiratory muscles of the airways (eg, tongue and pharyngeal muscles) and ribcage (eg, diaphragm and intercostal muscles). Similar to its actions on preBötC, binding of the neurotransmitter glutamate to AMPA receptors is a major contributor to the synaptic activation of respiratory motoneurons.[56,58,60,61] The amplitude of inspiratory drive transmitted to respiratory motoneurons can also be suppressed by opioids.

Ampakines are a class of synthetic compounds initially designed to enhance glutamatergic neurotransmission related to cognition, learning, and memory.[62–64] As demonstrated in initial early-stage clinical trials related to cognitive and affective disorders, ampakines are metabolically stable, readily cross the blood-brain barrier, and produce minimal side effects at therapeutic doses. The ampakine molecule itself does not directly activate AMPA receptors. Rather, ampakines interact in a highly specific manner with the AMPA receptor, lowering the amount of neurotransmitter required to generate a response, and increasing the magnitude and/or duration of the response to any given amount of glutamate (ie, they are positive allosteric modulators of AMPA receptors).

It was the combination of these features of ampakines with the fact that AMPA receptor activation is a key component of respiratory neural control that provided the foundation for the hypothesis that ampakines may counter respiratory depression induced by a multitude of pathogenic mechanisms and classes of drugs that cause hypoventilation.

Preclinical Rodent Data Demonstrating the Efficacy of Ampakines for Countering Opioid-Induced Respiratory Depression

The first testing of the hypothesis that ampakines would counter opioid-induced respiratory depression was carried out using in vitro perinatal rat preparations. This initial screening was followed with in vivo whole-body plethysmographic recordings from unanesthetized rats.

In Vitro Rodent Studies

The neonatal brainstem-spinal cord preparations have been well-characterized and shown to generate complex, coordinated patterns of respiratory-related activity.[65,66] Recordings from cervical ventral and hypoglossal cranial roots provide information regarding the pharmacology of respiratory rhythm generating networks and the pathways transmitting that respiratory drive to key output components of the respiratory motor system, without the confounding influence of peripheral chemoreceptors and supramedullary structures. The medullary slice preparation is a derivative of the brainstem-spinal cord preparation.[67] It contains the minimum component of neuronal populations within the ventrolateral medulla necessary for generating a respiratory rhythm, the preBötC. The medullary slice also contains a significant portion of the rostral ventral respiratory group, hypoglossal nucleus, and XII cranial nerve rootlets from which inspiratory motor discharge is recorded.

These in vitro models were initially used to examine the ability of the ampakines CX546 and CX717 to counter the depression of respiratory frequency and amplitude caused by the μ-opiate receptor agonist, D-Ala^2, N-MePhe^4, Gly-ol^5 (DAMGO).[49,50] Bath or focal applications of DAMGO into the preBötC caused a slowing and eventual cessation of respiratory rhythm, which was alleviated by subsequent application of ampakines either to the bathing medium or to focal injections into the preBötC. The preparations were also amenable for examining XII motoneuron activity. Most inspiratory synaptic transmissions to XII motoneurons, at least in vitro, are via glutamate acting through AMPA receptors.[58] Thus, the efficacy of ampakines to counter depressed inspiratory drive was tested. Consistent with what is observed within the preBötC, ampakines markedly reduced the DAMGO-induced suppression of XII motoneuron activity.[68]

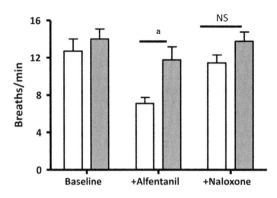

Fig. 6. Preadministration of the ampakine CX717 (1500 mg, oral) countered the decrease in respiratory frequency induced by alfentanil in human subjects (n = 15). [a] $P<.01$. NS, not significant. (*Adapted from* Oertel BG, Felden L, Tran PV, et al. Selective antagonism of opioid-induced respiratory depression by an AMPAKINE molecule in humans without loss of opioid analgesia. Clin Pharmacol Ther 2010;87:204–11; with permission.)

In Vivo Rodent Studies

Plethysmographic recordings were made from young and adult rats in which moderate to life-threatening apnea had been induced by varying doses of fentanyl administered either intraperitoneally or intravenously.[49,50] For each animal, an ampakine (CX546 or C717) was given either before or after the administration of fentanyl. Prophylactic administration of ampakine either before or concomitant with fentanyl markedly reduced respiratory depression. Furthermore, the administration of ampakine after the animals received a potentially lethal dose of fentanyl successfully rescued them from certain death.

Translational Human Data Demonstrating the Efficacy of Ampakines for Countering Opioid-Induced Respiratory Depression

A subsequent phase IIa clinical trial translated the rodent studies into man, showing that administration of an ampakine (CX717) can attenuate opioid-induced respiratory depression while leaving the analgesic effect intact (**Fig. 6**).[55] A double-blind, randomized crossover design study was conducted using the effect of an infusion of an opioid (alfentanil) on respiration and the response to a noxious stimulus to test for a prophylactic rescue action of the ampakine CX717. This ampakine, administered before testing, prevents the opioid-induced depression of respiratory rate and partially reverses the blunted response to CO_2 challenge without any effect on heat pain tolerance.

In summary, the preclinical and clinical studies demonstrated that ampakines counter opioid-induced respiratory depression while having the following favorable attributes: (i) ampakines do not alter the baseline sensitivity to painful stimuli in control animals; (ii) analgesia is preserved; (iii) therapeutic doses of ampakines do not alter baseline breathing (ie, induce hyperventilation under eupneic conditions). The underlying mechanism accounting for the fortuitous selective activation of depressed versus normative respiratory drive has not been determined.

Additional Applications of Ampakines for Alleviating Respiratory Depression

PreBötC neurons and respiratory motoneurons also express GABA (γ-aminobutyric acid) receptors, and thus respiratory depression can be induced by agents activating those receptors. These agents include propofol and the combination of pentobarbital and alcohol. Preclinical rodent data have demonstrated that ampakines are effective for countering respiratory depression induced by those agents.[51,52] Ampakines also alleviate weak endogenous respiratory drive in rodent models of apnea of prematurity[53] and Pompe disease.[54] This broad spectrum of ampakine efficacy arises from the fact that the molecular target, AMPA receptors, plays such a pivotal role in respiratory rhythmogenesis and inspiratory drive transmission to motoneurons. There are ongoing preclinical studies that are providing the foundation for yet further widening the therapeutic potential for ampakine therapy in the context of respiratory depression.

SUMMARY

Central apneas are frequent polysomnographic findings in patients with HF and those using opioids chronically for pain. A large number of studies have demonstrated that the presence of CSAs is associated with excess mortality in patients with HF, and ASV devices are quite helpful. However, the recent SERVE-HF trial casts doubt on this notion; however, there potential flaws in the trial and the fact that the discontinued, older generation ASV ventilator was used in the study. The new generation ASV devices have undergone major improvements in their algorithms, and the field anxiously awaits the results of the ADVENT-HF trial, which is in progress.

Chronic opioid use is an established risk factor for CSA. CSA may be present on initial diagnostic polysomnography or may emerge with initiation of CPAP therapy, referred to as opioid-associated complex sleep apnea. The first approach to therapy is to taper opioid use if possible. New generation servo ventilators and bilevel devices in the ST mode deserve further research, and the authors recommend them for treatment of CSA induced by chronic opioid use. The alternative of using the pharmacologic approach of ampakine administration warrants evaluation. The efficacy of ampakines to counter multiple types of central apnea in animal models, their safety profile, and several hour half-life supports their potential.

REFERENCES

1. Javaheri S, Dempsey JA. Central sleep apnea. Compr Physiol 2013;3:141–63.
2. Javaheri S. Heart failure. In: Kryger MH, Roth T, Dement WC, editors. Principles and practices of sleep medicine. 6th edition. Philadelphia: WB Saunders, in press.
3. Dowdell WT, Javaheri S, McGinnis W. Cheyne-Stokes respiration presenting as sleep apnea syndrome. Clinical and polysomnographic features. Am Rev Respir Dis 1990;141:871–9.
4. Javaheri S, Sands SA, Edwards BA. Acetazolamide attenuates Hunter-Cheyne-Stokes breathing yet paradoxically augments the hypercapnic ventilatory response in patients with heart failure. Ann Am Thorac Soc 2014;11:80–6.
5. Khayat R, Abraham W, Patt B, et al. Central sleep apnea is a predictor of cardiac readmission in hospitalized patients with systolic heart failure. J Cardiol 2012;18:534–40.
6. Javaheri S, Shukla R, Zeigler H, et al. Central sleep apnea, right ventricular dysfunction and low diastolic blood pressure are predictors of mortality in systolic heart failure. J Am Coll Cardiol 2007;49: 2028–34.
7. Javaheri S, Caref B, Chen E, et al. Sleep apnea testing and outcomes in a large cohort of Medicare beneficiaries with newly diagnosed heart failure. Am J Respir Crit Care Med 2011;183:539–46.
8. Bitter T, Faber L, Hering D, et al. Sleep-disordered breathing in heart failure with normal left ventricular ejection fraction. Eur J Heart Fail 2009;11:602–8.
9. Herrscher TE, Akre H, Øverland B, et al. High prevalence of sleep apnea in heart failure outpatients: even in patients with preserved systolic function. J Card Fail 2011;17:420–5.
10. Khayat R, Jarjoura D, Patt B, et al. In-hospital testing for sleep-disordered breathing in hospitalized

patients with decompensated heart failure: report of prevalence and patient characteristics. J Card Fail 2009;15(9):739–46.
11. Javaheri S. Heart failure. In: Kushida CA, editor. The encyclopedia of sleep, vol. 3. Waltham (MA): Academic Press; 2013. p. 374–86.
12. Javaheri S, Brown L, Randerath W. Positive airway pressure therapy with adaptive servo-ventilation (part II: clinical applications). Chest 2014;146:855–68.
13. Javaheri S, Abraham WT, Brown C, et al. Prevalence of obstructive sleep apnea and periodic limb movement in 45 subjects with heart transplantation. Eur Heart J 2004;25:260–6.
14. Ponikowski P, Javaheri S, Michalkiewicz D, et al. Transvenous phrenic nerve stimulation for the treatment of central sleep apnoea in heart failure. Eur Heart J 2012;33:889–94.
15. Bradley T, Logan A, Kimoff J, et al. Continuous positive airway pressure for central sleep apnea and heart failure. N Engl J Med 2006;353:2025–33.
16. Javaheri S. CPAP should not be used for central sleep apnea in congestive heart failure patients. J Clin Sleep Med 2006;2:399–402.
17. Javaheri S. Effects of continuous positive airway pressure on sleep apnea and ventricular irritability in patients with heart failure. Circulation 2000;101: 392–7.
18. Arzt M, Floras JS, Logan AG, et al. Suppression of central sleep apnea by continuous positive airway pressure and transplant-free survival in heart failure. A post-hoc analysis of the Canadian Continuous Positive Airway Pressure for patients with central sleep apnea and heart failure trial (CANPAP). Circulation 2007;115:3173–80.
19. Ryan CM, Floras JS, Logan AG, et al. Shift in sleep apnoea type in heart failure patients in the CANPAP trial. Eur Respir J 2010;35:592–7.
20. Javaheri S, Brown L, Randerath W. Positive airway pressure therapy with adaptive servoventilation (part 1: operational algorithms). Chest 2014;146: 514–23.
21. Brown LK, Javaheri S. Adaptive servoventilation for the treatment of central sleep apnea in congestive heart failure: what have we learned? Curr Opin Pulm Med 2014;20:550–7.
22. Sogol J, Shahrokh J. Nocturnal noninvasive ventilation in heart failure. In: Basner RC, Parthasarathy S, editors. Nocturnal non-invasive ventilation: theory, evidence, and practice. New York: Springer Science; 2015. p. 73–81.
23. Randerath WJ, Javaheri S. Adaptive servo-ventilation in central sleep apnea. Sleep Med Clin 2014;9:69–85.
24. Cowie MR, Woehrle H, Wegscheider K, et al. Adaptive servo-ventilation for central sleep apnea in systolic heart failure. N Engl J Med 2015;373(12):1095–105.
25. Ramar K, Ramar P, Morgenthaler TI. Adaptive servo-ventilation in patients with central or complex sleep

apnea related to chronic opioid use and congestive heart failure. J Clin Sleep Med 2012;8(5):569–76.

26. Zhang XL, Ding N, Wang H, et al. Transvenous phrenic nerve stimulation in patients with Cheyne-Stokes respiration and congestive heart failure—a safety and proof-of-concept study. Chest 2012; 142:927–34.

27. Zhang XL, Ding N, Ni B, et al. Safety and feasibility of chronic transvenous phrenic nerve stimulation for the treatment of central sleep apnea in heart failure patients. Clin Respir J 2015. http://dx.doi.org/10.1111/crj. 12320.

28. Abraham WT, Jagielski D, Oldenburg O, et al, On behalf of the remedē® Pilot Study Investigators. Phrenic nerve stimulation for the treatment of central sleep apnea. JACC Heart Fail 2015;5:360–9.

29. Costanzo MR, Augostini R, Goldberg LR, et al. Design of the remedē® system pivotal trial: a prospective, randomized study in the use of respiratory rhythm management to treat central sleep apnea. J Card Fail 2015;21(11):892–902.

30. Joranson DE, Ryan KM, Gilson AM, et al. Trends in medical use abuse of opioid analgesics. JAMA 2000;283(13):1710–4.

31. ARCOS. Automation of reports and consolidated orders system, editor. Retail drug summary. US Department of Justice; DEA; 2005.

32. Monitoring the future (MTF) survey, US. Services DoHaH; 2005.

33. Unintentional drug poisoning in the United States. National Center for Injury Prevention and Control CfDCaP; 2010.

34. Centers for Disease Control and Prevention (CDC). Increase in poisoning deaths caused by non-illicit drugs—Utah 1991-2003. MMWR Morb Mortal Wkly Rep 2005;54:3–6.

35. Javaheri S, Malik A, Smith J, et al. Adaptive pressure support servoventilation: a novel treatment for sleep apnea associated with use of opioids. J Clin Sleep Med 2008;4(4):305–10.

36. Javaheri S, Harris N, Howard J, et al. Adaptive servo-ventilation for treatment of opioids-associated central sleep apnea. J Clin Sleep Med 2014;10:637–43.

37. Webster LR, Choi Y, Desai H, et al. Sleep-disordered breathing and chronic opioid therapy. Pain Med 2008;9(4):425–32.

38. Teichtahl H, Prodromidis A, Miller B, et al. Sleep-disordered breathing in stable methadone programme patients: a pilot study. Addiction 2001; 96(3):395–403.

39. Farney RJ, Walker JM, Cloward TV, et al. Sleep-disordered breathing associated with long-term opioid therapy. Chest 2003;123(2):632–9.

40. Farney RJ, Walker JM, Boyle KM, et al. Adaptive servoventilation (ASV) in patients with sleep disordered breathing associated with chronic opioid medications for non-malignant pain. J Clin Sleep Med 2008;4(4):311–9.

41. Javaheri S, Cao M. Opioid induced central sleep apnea. In: Fabiani M, editor. Proceedings of the X World Congress on sleep apnea, section: respiratory disorders and snoring. Turin (Italy): Edizioni Minerva Medica; 2012. p. 133–7.

42. Cao M, Javaheri S. Chronic opioid use: effects on respiration and sleep. In: Tvildiani D, Gegechkori K, editors. Opioids pharmacology, clinical uses and adverse effects. New York: Nova Science Publishers, Inc; 2012. p. 1–13.

43. Arora N, Cao M, Javaheri S. Opioids, sedatives, and sleep hypoventilation. Sleep Med Clin 2014;9:391–8.

44. Javaheri S, Smith J, Chung J. The prevalence and natural history of complex sleep apnea. J Clin Sleep Med 2009;5:205–11.

45. Allam JS, Olson EJ, Gay PC, et al. Efficacy of adaptive servoventilation in treatment of complex and central sleep apnea syndromes. Chest 2007; 132(6):1839–46.

46. Cao M, Cardell CY, Willes L, et al. A novel adaptive servoventilation (ASVAuto) for the treatment of central sleep apnea associated with chronic use of opioids. J Clin Sleep Med 2014; 10(8):855–61.

47. Troitino A, Labedi N, Kufel T, et al. Positive airway pressure therapy in patients with opioid-related central sleep apnea. Sleep Breath 2014;18:367–73.

48. Guilleminault C, Cao M, Yue HJ, et al. Obstructive sleep apnea and chronic opioid use. Lung 2010; 188(6):459–68.

49. Ren J, Poon BY, Tang Y, et al. Ampakines alleviate respiratory depression in rats. Am J Respir Crit Care Med 2006;174:1384–91.

50. Ren J, Ding X, Funk GD, et al. Ampakine CX717 protects against fentanyl-induced respiratory depression and lethal apnea in rats. Anesthesiology 2009;110:1364–70.

51. Ren J, Ding X, Greer JJ. Respiratory depression in rats induced by alcohol and barbiturate and alleviation by ampakine CX717. J Appl Physiol (1985) 2012;113(7):1004–11.

52. Ren J, Lenal F, Yang M, et al. Co-administration of the ampakine CX717 with propofol reduces respiratory depression and fatal apneas. Anesthesiology 2013;118(6):1437–45.

53. Ren J, Ding X, Greer JJ. Ampakines enhance weak endogenous respiratory drive and apnea in perinatal rats. Am J Respir Crit Care Med 2015; 191(6):704–10.

54. El Mallah MK, Pagliardini S, Turner SM, et al. Stimulation of respiratory motor output and ventilation in a murine model of Pompe disease by ampakines. Am J Respir Cell Mol Biol 2015;53(3):326–35.

55. Oertel BG, Felden L, Tran PV, et al. Selective antagonism of opioid-induced respiratory depression by

an AMPAKINE molecule in humans without loss of opioid analgesia. Clin Pharmacol Ther 2010;87: 204–11.

56. Greer JJ, Smith JC, Feldman JL. The role of excitatory amino acids in the generation and transmission of respiratory drive in the neonatal rat. J Physiol 1991;1001(437):727–49.

57. Ge Q, Feldman JL. AMPA receptor activation and phosphatase inhibition affect neonatal rat respiratory rhythm generation. J Physiol 1998;509:255–66.

58. Funk GD, Smith JC, Feldman JL. Generation and transmission of respiratory oscillations in medullary slices: role of excitatory amino acids. J Neurophysiol 1993;70:1497–515.

59. Pace RW, Mackay DD, Feldman JL, et al. Inspiratory bursts in the preBötzinger complex depend on a calcium-activated non-specific cation current linked to glutamate receptors in neonatal mice. J Physiol 2007;582:113–25.

60. Liu G, Feldman JL, Smith JC. Excitatory amino acid-mediated transmission of inspiratory drive to phrenic motoneurons. J Neurophysiol 1990;64:423–36.

61. Chitravanshi VC, Sapru HN. NMDA as well as non-NMDA receptors mediate the neurotransmission of inspiratory drive to phrenic motoneurons in the adult rat. Brain Res 1996;715(1–2):104–12.

62. Lynch G. Glutamate-based therapeutic approaches: ampakines. Curr Opin Pharmacol 2006;6:82–8.

63. Lynch G, Gall CM. Ampakines and the threefold path to cognitive enhancement. Trends Neurosci 2006;29(10):554–62.

64. Arai AC, Xia YF, Suzuki E. Modulation of AMPA receptor kinetics differentially influences synaptic plasticity in the hippocampus. Neuroscience 2004; 123:1011–24.

65. Greer JJ, Smith JC, Feldman JL. Generation of respiratory and locomotor patterns by an in vitro brainstem-spinal cord fetal rat preparation. J Neurophysiol 1992;67:996–9.

66. Smith JC, Greer JJ, Liu G, et al. Neural mechanisms generating respiratory pattern in mammalian brainstem-spinal cord in vitro. I. Spatiotemporal patterns of motor and medullary neuron activity. J Neurophysiol 1990;64:1149–69.

67. Smith JC, Ellenberger HH, Ballanyi K, et al. PreBötzinger complex: a brainstem region that may generate respiratory rhythm in mammals. Science 1991;1001(254):726–9.

68. Lorier AL, Funk GL, Greer JJ. Opiate-induced suppression of rat hypoglossal motoneuron activity and its reversal by ampakine therapy. PLoS One 2010;5(1):e8766.

The Role of Big Data in the Management of Sleep-Disordered Breathing

Rohit Budhiraja, MD[a,b], Robert Thomas, MD, MMSc[c],
Matthew Kim, MD[d], Susan Redline, MD, MPH[e,f],*

KEYWORDS

- Sleep-disordered breathing • Big data • Management • Sleep apnea

KEY POINTS

- Analysis of large-volume data holds the promise for improving the application of precision medicine to sleep, including improving the identification of patient subgroups who may specifically benefit from alternative therapies.
- Big data used within the health care system also promises to facilite end-to-end screening, diagnosis, and management of sleep disorders; improve the recognition of differences in presentation and susceptibility to sleep apnea; and lead to improved management and outcomes.
- To meet the vision of personalized, precision therapeutics and diagnostics and improving the efficiciency and quality of sleep medicine will require ongoing efforts, investments, and some change in our current medical and research cultures.
- Expanding electronic health records with well-defined sleep data and further development and growth of national research repositories and patient networks and registries are important strategies for achieving these goals.
- Any successful strategy will need to integrate patient-collected data through the rapidly evolving wearable device market.

INTRODUCTION

Despite considerable investments in health care, our health care systems often fall short in meeting quality metrics, patient satisfaction, and clinical outcomes goals.[1] Furthermore, despite large investments in clinical research, our research infrastructure often does not yield the needed data to support evidence-based health care. Deficiencies are partially due to inadequate representation of key stakeholders, including patients, in the design of health care research as well as due to the overall paucity of valid and comprehensive data on sufficient numbers of patients. These gaps are especially evident in sleep medicine, whereby data are lacking that address questions, such as which patients benefit from alternative treatments (eg,

Support in part by NIH R24HL114473 and Patient-Centered Outcomes Research Institute PPRN-1306-04344.
[a] Division of Sleep and Circadian Disorders, Brigham and Women's Hospital, Harvard Medical School, Boston, MA, USA; [b] Division of Pulmonary and Critical Care Medicine, Department of Medicine, Brigham and Women's Hospital, Harvard Medical School, Boston, MA, USA; [c] Division of Pulmonary, Critical Care & Sleep Medicine, Department of Medicine, Beth Israel Deaconess Medical Center, Harvard Medical School, 330 Brookline Avenue, Boston, MA, USA; [d] Division of Endocrinology, Diabetes and Hypertension, Department of Medicine, Brigham and Women's Hospital, Harvard Medical School, Boston, MA, USA; [e] Division of Sleep and Circadian Disorders, Brigham and Women's Hospital, Harvard Medical School, 221 Longwood Avenue, Boston, MA 02115, USA; [f] Division of Pulmonary, Critical Care & Sleep Medicine, Department of Medicine, Beth Israel Deaconess Medical Center, Harvard Medical School, 330 Brookline Avenue, Boston, MA 02215, USA
* Corresponding author.
E-mail address: sredline@partners.org

Sleep Med Clin 11 (2016) 241–255
http://dx.doi.org/10.1016/j.jsmc.2016.01.009
1556-407X/16/$ – see front matter © 2016 Elsevier Inc. All rights reserved.

continuous positive airway pressure [CPAP], surgery, oral appliances, oxygen supplementation); the basis for interindividual variation in cardiometabolic and cognitive effects of sleep apnea; and the individual determinants of CPAP adherence or residual sleepiness after CPAP treatment. These gaps are due to limitations of available data, which too often are inadequate to generate robust evidence for supporting health care decisions. There is simultaneously a richness of data (eg, compliance tracking) and data waste (eg, focusing on insurance payments requirements while discarding other available data). The traditional practice of generating data has been compared with working in silos. Data silos include those such as electronic medical records of clinical encounters, sleep laboratory databases, and online positive airway pressure (PAP) tracking databases that reside in independent noncommunicating areas.

Although the strength of evidence depends on the validity and reliability of the data used to generate that evidence, with all other things being similar, a larger n yields comparatively superior evidence with higher statistical power and a lower likelihood of erroneous inferences. Small-sized studies may be difficult to reproduce. Indeed, it has been suggested that most published studies cannot be replicated.[2] The current health care model uses data from studies conducted on hundreds or possibly thousands of people to determine the recommendations for millions of people. Information is typically generated based on data from one or a few clinical centers and is often limited in diversity of patient representation, environmental backgrounds, and practice variation. The understudied and underserved populations are also at a risk of inappropriate therapy based on using data from studies performed on majority cohorts. The use of data from single or a few centers also does not provide the statistical power to provide evidentiary information about individual variation in clinical response or risk specific to given individuals. Rather, inferences often only address average effects (in the sampled population), and the datasets are underpowered to detect differences that may be relevant to smaller subgroups of individuals.

The widespread use of electronic health record (EHR) systems and advances in computational power and analytical methods provide new opportunities to amass data of unprecedented size, heterogeneity, and complexity and analyze these with new analytical methods, thus, overcoming the gaps described earlier. *Big data* refers to voluminous databases that allow exploration of the effects of individual differences and complex interactions with the goal of facilitating identification and management of individuals according to their unique characteristics (ie, personalizing medicine or pursuing precision medicine). Big data can be defined by 3 *Vs*: volume, velocity, and variety. The *volume* or the size of the data underlines the appeal and the value of the database. Generally, the bigger the size of the dataset, the higher the statistical power for analyses and ability to drill down to analysis of subgroups and to reduce the likelihood of making spurious inferences. *Velocity* is the rate at which the data are generated and analyzed. Modern devices, such as smartphones, generate data almost in real time, which can lead to remarkably quick discoveries, quantifying dynamic changes in a population's health, such as improving recognition of newly emergent food-borne or infectious disease outbreaks. Finally, *variety* refers to different sources, types, and formats of data. They may be obtained from social media, disease-oriented Web sites (such as MyApnea.org),[3] smartphones, medical records, or a combination of all these. Thus, in considering big data, one needs to consider the sample size of available data, the dimensionality of those data, the access to those data, and the analytical and computational resources used to maximize information from the data.

A major source of big data is from the EHR, which has the power to transform each patient encounter as a datum in a potentially massive longitudinal database. There are efforts to expand the EHR to contain more comprehensive and searchable fields of routinely collected clinical data as well as to incorporate and link data from external sources, such as from validated patient surveys, health devices, and even genomic data. The ability to search multiple well-annotated medical notes, laboratory values, imaging studies, biomarkers, and data regarding progression of disease offers the prospect of using knowledge from massive interconnected databases from large numbers of patients to guide therapy to an individual patient, improve public health, and enhance quality of care in general. Recognizing this potential, in addition to the challenges of accessing and integrating sleep data into the EHR, the American Academy of Sleep Medicine organized a task force to begin the process of specifying EHR needs in sleep medicine (see Hwang D: Monitoring Progress and Adherence with Positive Airway Pressure Therapy for Obstructive Sleep Apnea: The Roles of Telemedicine and Mobile Health Applications, in this issue).

The widespread collection of data during routine daily activities through mobile phones, wearables, and other devices provides opportunities to nonintrusively extract real-time data from multiple sources, integrating these with research and clinical datasets. These data are of high relevance to sleep medicine, whereby measures of sleep patterns, snoring, and PAP adherence are available through mobile devices.

Big data have the potential to fast track scientific advancement in medicine by linking the omics data (genomics, metabolomics, proteomics, expression, and so forth), molecular biology, clinical data, population data, and mobile data, among others, to understand the diverse aspects of disorders and to facilitate personalized management. These goals are tightly linked to establishing precision medicine as a goal for health care of the future. Supported by the National Institutes of Health (NIH), the US Veteran's Administration (VA), and other national and international organizations, precision medicine initiatives support activities leading to the use of multiple sources of patient-specific information (genomic, clinical, behavioral, environmental, and patient preference) to identify and apply customized health care decisions, practices, and products that meet individual patient needs. Moving away from models of care that focus on a population's average response but often result in suboptimal treatment for many, precision medicine seeks to use big data to identify which treatments result in favorable responses, optimize safety and reduce harm, and improve long-term health outcomes for *specific* individuals. Although still nascent, notable progress has been made in tailoring therapies for patients with cancer, thrombotic diseases, immunologic disorders, among others; these examples provide models for sleep medicine.

It is useful to conceptualize levels or strata of big data in sleep sciences and sleep medicine. These levels include *population-level information* from multiple representative samples across the world composed of individuals not usually specifically selected for disease; *disease specific information*, composed of data on patients ascertained by diseases (eg, narcolepsy, sleep apnea, insomnia) and; *individual-level information*, now increasingly enabled through point-of-care longitudinal data tracking and including information, such as body weight, blood glucose, blood pressure, and from wearable devices.

The following sections discuss the potential of big data in providing insights into the pathophysiology, presentation, and management of sleep-disordered breathing (SDB) and for approaches for sleep precision medicine.

CAUSE AND GENETIC PREDISPOSITION

Developing pharmacologic interventions for sleep apnea has been limited by insufficient understanding of its specific cause and limitations of current phenotyping strategies. The pathogenesis of sleep apnea likely involves complex interactions between genetic factors that influence anatomy and pharyngeal neuromuscular control, sleep fragmentation propensity, respiratory chemoreflex activation, and environmental exposures. For more than 20 years it has been known that sleep apnea aggregates within families and that the apnea hypopnea index (AHI) has significant heritability,[4,5] defined as the portion of the trait variance attributable to familial, and typically genetic, influences. Although obesity is a significant risk factor for sleep apnea, approximately 60% of the genetic basis for sleep apnea is through body mass index–independent pathways,[6] suggesting the potential for novel intervention targets. Early studies of the molecular genetics of sleep apnea were limited to modest-sized association studies of candidate genes that identified several genetic variants to be associated with the AHI,[7,8] but results were largely not replicated in independent samples. Recent efforts to aggregate larger amounts of sleep phenotype and genotype data from NIH-funded cohorts have identified additional putative loci (Cade; in press), which also await independent replication. Even the latter efforts, representing the world's largest sleep apnea genetic database and interactions among international centers (International Sleep Genetic Epidemiology Consortium; sleepgenetics.org), have analyzed genotype and phenotype data for less than 25,000 individuals. Although this sample is large for clinical trials or epidemiologic studies, it is estimated to be only one-tenth the size needed to identify rare genetic variants. Furthermore, given that genetic architecture varies by ancestry and analysis of multiethnic samples can accelerate variant discovery, newer approaches are needed to achieve both the sample sizes as well as the racial/ethnic diversity to identify and validate functional variants. Because of the rapid reduction in genotyping costs, lack of genotypes is no longer a barrier to genetic discovery. Rather, there is a 2-fold big data need: (1) to link sleep apnea cases from the EHR to genetic samples and (2) to identify sleep phenotypes that are both scalable across large samples and informative. The former need may be addressed through NIH and VA investments in initiatives, such as the Million Veteran Program,[9] Electronic Medical Records and Genomics,[10] and NIH Precision Medicine Cohorts, with each program aiming to deposit genotype data within the EHR. The challenge for sleep medicine is to ensure that the appropriate clinical data on sleep disorders are captured and are extractable within the EHR so that they can be linked to these genetic resources. The second need is to improve the sleep phenotype data within research cohorts with genetic data, including efforts to capture relevant and easily measured sleep phenotypes on large numbers of individuals. Such improvement may be incumbent upon moving beyond the AHI as the key metric for sleep apnea genetics. In addition to not providing information on attributes of sleep apnea that may reflect intermediate pathways, measurement of the AHI can be burdensome. Furthermore, recent research indicates that alternative sleep apnea measurements, such as the average apnea hypopnea duration and average nocturnal oxygen saturation, have higher heritability than the AHI, with even greater heritability achieved by combining information from multiple sleep apnea traits as principal components (Wang, in press). Therefore, big data to promote the discovery of sleep apnea susceptibility genes and related molecular pathways require further integration of clinical sleep data within the EHR as well as collection of informative and scalable phenotypes in large research cohorts.

Genes likely influence not only the causation of sleep apnea but also the complications thereof. Although factors, such as oxidative stress and endothelial dysfunction, account for the pathogenesis of several complications of this disorder,[11] it is possible that a genetic susceptibility may be required for certain complications: a 2-hit mechanism. For example, sleep apnea is associated with 5 times greater odds of risk of cognitive impairment in women with the apolipoprotein E (ApoE) epsilon4 allele, but no significant increase is encountered in women with sleep apnea lacking this allele.[12] Other studies confirm the worse cognitive function in ApoE epsilon4-positive individuals with sleep apnea than those without this allele.[13,14] It may be hypothesized that sleep apnea–related hypoxemia, inflammation, and oxidative stress impacts brain function most severely in those with genetic susceptibility to cognitive disorders. A large repository of genetic and neurophysiologic markers of sleep apnea can conceivably help predict the vulnerability to complications as well as the likelihood of benefit from sleep interventions.

Finally, there is shared heritability of sleep apnea with other traits, including obesity and diabetes. Big data efforts, which bring multiple phenotypes together, can further identify shared genetic pathways as well as help identify additional predictors of health and disease. Identification of phenotypic and genetic markers will help understand the genetic basis and heritability of sleep apnea as well as related disorders and might help identify novel therapeutic targets that address multiple disease pathways.

DIAGNOSIS

Polysomnography (PSG) is the current gold standard for diagnosing sleep apnea but suffers from several shortcomings. The current metric to quantify sleep apnea is the AHI. However, it is an imperfect predictor of symptoms and adverse health outcomes. Furthermore, apneas and hypopneas can be defined in many different ways (based on amplitude changes, desaturations, and arousals), with limited data on the association between different definitions, symptoms, and outcomes.[15] Several different sensors are available for determining the magnitude of change in flow and effort, and may yield variable AHI values.[15,16] Finally, phenomena like flow limitation and rapid eye movement–related sleep apnea may have symptomatic and outcome implications but are not recognized by many health insurance providers because of the lack of substantial data demonstrating their clinical significance.[17]

The traditional PSG interpretation does not routinely include quantitative analysis and reporting of potentially important metrics of physiologic function, such as sleep assessment with electroencephalography (EEG) power spectral analyses and heart rate variability analysis.[18] Accumulation, aggregation, and analysis of neurologic and cardiorespiratory data could yield superior metrics for diagnosing the sleep apnea syndrome and improving the management; however, a role for these more complex metrics requires systematic assessments of their independent prediction or ability to discriminate important subgroups of the population. Although genetic and clinical specimen databases, such as the National Heart, Lung, and Blood Institute's (NHLBI's) Biologic Specimen and Data Repository Information Coordinating Center allow linking biological and genetic specimen information with clinical data and promote research, there are few repositories for polysomnographic variables and sleep study data (see resources section).[19] PhysioNet (physionet.org) is a Web resource for several databases with diverse signals, including electrocardiogram (ECG), continuous invasive blood pressure, respiration, oxygen saturation, EEG, interbeat (RR) interval databases, gait and balance databases, neuroelectric and myoelectric data, and magnetic resonance angiography images.[20,21] As described later, the National Sleep Research Resource (NSRR) (sleepdata.org) is an NIH-funded research repository that could be used to develop and test new quantitative sleep algorithms, which might then be applied to clinical records. To maximize the use of clinical PSG information, there needs to be further efforts at standardizing not only the collection but also the annotation and storage of the volumes of clinical PSGs performed each year. As discussed earlier, such data, when linked to other EHR data and potential deposits of genomic data, could provide fertile ground for developing better metrics for disease screening, diagnosis, and prediction.

Mobile fitness trackers promise another rich source of germane data. Sleep duration, physical activity, and calorie intake are important factors that can lead to the genesis or progression of sleep apnea or the complications thereof. However, clinicians rarely query patients in details regarding these lifestyle variables during clinical encounters. Even when the patients are asked, their replies may not be sufficiently specific or may be limited by recall bias. The smartphones and wrist sensors now collect a bevy of health data, and the application designers continue to make the application software more sophisticated with increasingly valid and reliable data collection. Use of such data can provide objective information about factors, including diet, physical activity, and sleep duration, which can influence the severity of sleep apnea and symptoms, including sleepiness. The applications can also help provide frequent visual feedback to patients and promote healthy behaviors. They can significantly assist management of SDB; education regarding these behaviors is an integral, albeit sometimes overlooked, part of therapy. With validation, these applications can play a role in screening for SDB. Wearable devices can also provide information on night-to-night variability of abnormality. Phenotyping of sleep quality during sleep apnea therapy and detecting persistence of periodic breathing and central apneas can be detected using wearable devices (eg, M1,[22] S+[23]). There is ongoing interest in how such devices can be integrated into the EHR and used for clinical care, especially given that they are not currently designed to meet clear specifications (eg, by Food and Drug Administration or professional societies).

The risk stratification of people who present with sleep complaints is based on identification of key symptoms or presenting signs, often collected by questionnaires. Existing screening questionnaires have been developed using data that reflect average patients with sleep apnea, who often are middle aged, male, and overweight. These questions are likely to have more limited utility in identifying important subgroups with sleep apnea, including individuals who are normal weight or underweight, women, and young or older adults. Big-volume data may allow better screening algorithms specific to individuals based on their gender, ethnicity, anatomy etc. Furthermore,

although questionnaires like the Epworth Sleepiness Scale[24,25] are widely used to assess daytime sleepiness, they only have a limited correlation with objective sleepiness measurements. Multiple sleep latency tests and multiple wakeful tests provide objective assessments of daytime sleepiness but are expensive, burdensome, and not commonly used. Use of big data to infer levels of alertness based on patterns of daily activities (eg, activity levels, vigilance) may provide novel opportunities to assess patient function and response to treatment with minimal patient burden. Continuous real-life collection of these data can provide more representative information than a one-time questionnaire or a 1-day objective study in an artificial environment.

MANAGEMENT

Big data may facilitate dynamic, accurate, and effective management of sleep disorders. Data from large EHR databases may help determine the best treatment of patients by evaluating therapy outcomes over time and comparing data in patients who are similar but who receive alternative treatments. This observational study design, although not as rigorous as a randomized controlled trial, can use techniques such as propensity score matching to provide valid inferences. Big data allow these propensity scores to be calculated reliably from large numbers of individuals. Use of multiple indices of disease risk and outcomes may also more accurately predict the chances of success of a therapy than the crude clinical estimates based on smaller numbers of variables. Effectively, millions of data points help create a multidimensional resource and allow more sophisticated pattern matching. Such an analysis would ask the following: What was the outcome when patients with the most similar characteristics and circumstances were managed in a particular manner? This question can also be framed to be patient centric by providing patients with information on how patients most similar to them fared with specific therapies. The strict eligibility criteria of most clinical trials exclude many patients seen in routine clinical practice. Having access to large-scale EHRs can help the broadest group of patients make more informed decisions regarding their management.

PAP is currently considered the treatment of choice for most patients with obstructive sleep apnea (OSA). Alternative therapies, including oral appliances, surgery, and positional therapies, are usually reserved for patients who fail PAP therapy. However, is PAP therapy indeed the optimum first-line therapy, no matter the unique characteristics and personal preferences of patients? Availability of big data would afford more reliable subgroup analyses, including use of data on patient preference, and, thence, facilitate a more individualized approach to managing OSA. Such insight will be instrumental in improving treatment adherence, effectiveness, and appropriate use of resources. Future decisions informed by big data could be based on algorithms using patients' anatomy, presentation, traditional and novel polysomnographic variables, biomarkers, imaging, genetics, and preferences. With better insight into what will likely work for patients, and initiating the right therapy at the right time, has potentially huge advantages over current predominantly heuristic approaches.

Comprehensive use of data from the EHR could help identify which interventions may be most beneficial for a particular patient and patients most similar to each given patient (based on the multiple factors enumerated earlier). Did such patients have better adherence with spousal support, psychological support, peer support, or other mediation? If so, similar interventions could be used to optimize CPAP therapy without having to embark on an ad hoc trial-and-error intervention. This intervention could significantly diminish the wasted time and effort for both the provider and patients and alleviate the disease, debility, and financial burden on the health care system. What are the nontraditional factors that contribute to poor adherence? Are the people who are less able to articulate or express themselves, for example, those with limited English or health literacy or with limited social support, at higher risk for nonadherence? Are they the ones who will likely not contact the health care system if there are any issues with management? How can the provider minimize the risks in these groups and improve the adherence? Access to sufficient and relevant data could facilitate such analyses.

Big data may also shed further light on the substantial issue of PAP therapy nonadherence. Currently, several factors have been suggested to be associated with CPAP adherence, but the current models of nonadherence explain only a small degree of variation in outcomes. Analysis of large samples and daily trends in PAP use may elucidate patterns that relate to what limits or promotes CPAP adherence. Better understanding of factors influencing adherence can help decide which patients to start on PAP therapy. For example, knowing if a given patient was nonadherent to asthma inhalers or hypertension medications might predict adherence to CPAP. Big data analyses could predict the likelihood of nonadherence based on multiple inputs, including past adherence behavior as well as patients'

age, sex, race, severity of sleep apnea, daytime symptoms, personality, and hundreds of other variables. This kind of analyses should be superior to a provider's empirical judgment, which usually takes into account only on a small subset of these factors and is limited by one's individual ability to integrate large amounts of information and potential personal biases. Ideally, such information would not replace the provider judgment or insight but enhance it and make it more precise and evidence based.

Big data may also improve the understanding of PAP adherence by providing dynamic feedback on factors that can be leveraged to improve adherence as well as offering the ability to individualize support. Smartphones provide continuous objective data over long periods rather than from a single point in time, often only at a clinic visit. For individuals, feedback on behaviors, such as steps walked, weight lifted, nutritional information, subjective sleep, mood, emotions, and so forth, could be correlated with the CPAP use the night before, help develop individual targets, and provide motivation for CPAP use. The feedback patients receive from their devices can also help them decide to seek help earlier before a pattern of nonadherence has been established.[26] Visualization and analysis of temporal patterns of use from PAP machines, even including nonwear time, would better describe actual CPAP patters and residual sleep apnea than current approaches that focus on simple summary measures (average hours per night). For example, a patient uses CPAP for 2 hours on one night and 6 hours the next. Based on the current payer requirements, a goal of an average of 4 hours a night would have been met; many providers may not further address important night-to-night variation in use. However, the patient might do much worse on the day following the 2-hour-use night and may be vulnerable to not only to the side effects of poor sleep, such as increased irritability, poor concentration, and lower productivity at home, but also to increased traffic accidents. Despite an arguably arbitrary cutoff of 4 hours of use for every patient, the definitions and consequences of underuse may vary significantly among different patients. Longitudinal estimation of total sleep time and residual apnea off PAP can enable calculation of the true residual untreated disease burden. The same principles are relevant to any sleep apnea treatment, including an oral appliance, weight loss, surgical approaches and body positioning. Models for tracking of sleep and breathing during sleep in home environments can be developed using approaches for blood pressure, weight, and home glucose monitoring.

Big data can be used not only to guide the management of sleep apnea but also to understand the geographic, regional, institutional, or even provider-level variations in outcomes. These data can be used for quality-improvement purposes and to direct educational resources toward specific providers to improve outcomes.

COMPLICATIONS OF OBSTRUCTIVE SLEEP APNEA

Sleep apnea is associated with several physiologic alterations, including hypoxia, inflammation, endothelial dysfunction, metabolic dysregulation, and sympathetic activation.[11] These alterations, along with genetic susceptibility, partly explain the association between OSA and diverse adverse consequences, including hypertension,[27–29] cardiovascular disease,[30–32] metabolic derangements,[28,33–35] neurologic changes,[36,37] and increased mortality.[37] However, several issues pertaining to these associations remain uncertain. It is yet unclear which patients will have which consequences. Studies with limited numbers of subjects have variably shown AHI, ODI, arousal index, time less than 88% oxygen saturation, and sleep architecture as polysomnographic predictors of consequences.[38] However, these metrics are not robust predictor of consequences. It also is unclear what demographic and clinical features suggest a worse outcome. Factors such as sleepiness and habitual short sleep duration may modify the risk of adverse outcomes with OSA and response to treatment.[39,40] Several studies suggest racial differences in the outcomes[35,41]; but whether race determines the consequences independent of multiple confounders, such as socioeconomic and environmental factors, is less clear. Similarly, there are sex-based differences in outcomes, which need further exploration and may be further influenced by age and cumulative years of sleep apnea exposure.[42]

Improved prediction of outcomes may be anticipated through better access and use of big data. Analyses of EHRs from millions of patients can provide higher power to detect the risk factors independently associated with diverse outcomes in patients with sleep apnea. It may be particularly informative to access longitudinal data to estimate years of exposure to OSA and consider how age of onset of sleep apnea, years of exposure, and timing of interventions all influence sleep apnea outcomes and treatment response. There is likely a large degree of individual variability in susceptibility to the various effects of sleep apnea, including differences in which organ systems may be most affected. It is unclear how such differences relate to differences in subtypes of sleep apnea (eg, associated with different degrees of hypoxemia or sleep fragmentation), duration of untreated disease, or to other underlying comorbidities, including obesity and diabetes or genetic variation. Only through access to very large data sets can patterns of risk be identified. This identification would require deep analysis of fully detailed sleep apnea data with data on demographics, clinical variables, and genetic factors.

Finally, there is the opportunity to better analyze big data for the purpose of better defining outcomes using online data sharing and crowdsourcing use of community wisdom to address a wide variety of challenges. A recent example was evident is a competition whereby algorithms designed by an audience registrant team predicted amyotrophic lateral sclerosis (ALS) disease progression better than a baseline algorithm as well as clinicians from top ALS clinics.[43] This competition also identified potential new predictors of disease progression, including creatinine and blood pressure. Using the NSRR, the community has interacted to help develop algorithms for detecting airflow limitation (sleepdata.org).

ASSOCIATIONS WITH OTHER DISORDERS

Voluminous databases with data variables encompassing several disorders offer the potential for studying the prevalence, presentation, and consequences of SDB in patients with diverse disorders. Several conditions, including but not limited to heart failure, stroke, renal disorders, pulmonary hypertension, idiopathic pulmonary fibrosis, Cushing syndrome, acromegaly, and Down syndrome, are associated with an increased prevalence of sleep apnea.[44–48] The risk factors, features, and consequences of sleep apnea in these conditions, especially the less common disorders, have not been adequately researched. The patients with some of these disorders may lack usual symptoms of sleep apnea, which may go undetected and untreated because of atypical presentations. Additionally, the direction of causality when sleep apnea is comorbid with diverse disorders is not always clear; SDB may result from pathophysiologic changes attributable to the primary disorders or it may contribute to their progression, and some of these associations may be bidirectional. However, limited data have impeded a better understanding of these relationships. Furthermore, the consequences of sleep apnea and its therapy on sleep quality, quality of life, and clinical progression of the comorbid disorders are unclear. Conversely, the effect of treatment of these disorders on prevalence of sleep apnea requires better definition.

Improved insights into the association of sleep apnea with these disorders, as feasible through big data, may not only facilitate improving outcomes in the primary disorders but may also shed more light on the pathophysiology of sleep apnea. One caveat is that although pooling of data will allow analyses of large numbers of patients even with rare disorders, several studies show that patients are rarely asked about their sleep symptoms unless they volunteer this information. Thus, there is a need to ensure that the sleep history is included as a standard part of history taking along with medical, social, and family history.

DEVELOPING BIG DATA RESOURCES

Relevant data for research and clinical sleep medicine are diverse and include data from overnight sleep recordings containing neuro-cardio-respiratory signals, PAP machines, patient-report outcome surveys, other clinical information, and biomarker and genetic data. Several steps can facilitate development of big data resources in sleep that yield valid inferences (**Box 1**). Identifying the best sources of such data and defining those data using structured approaches, such as defining the meta-data associated with each set of terms and measurements, enhances the ability to aggregate and analyze data from many sources. When possible, data from different sources should be harmonized to minimize the differences in the property being measured. This coordination serves to minimize random or misclassification and improve the ability to draw valid inferences.

In the absence of complete data standardization, several approaches to structuring and defining data can facilitate data curation, federation, integration, and analysis. *Metadata* is a standardized way of describing the data to facilitate location, retrieval, and utilization information. *Provenance* describes the origin of the data: the when, where, and how it was created. Provenance for sleep variables would specify the sensors used for data collection and how the data were scored and interpreted. Provenance allows the data to be tracked through various changes over time, such as occurs with sleep laboratory equipment replacements or new scoring standards. *Ontology* refers to a classification scheme, which describes the terms or concepts associated with specific data elements and shows how these elements relate to one another. It allows the implicit knowledge of the data to be characterized by specific logical properties and, thus, provides a framework for extracting and sharing data across users. *Domain ontologies* formalize and standardize the data language to overcome the semantic heterogeneity and create a machine-understandable specification of what exists in a given domain. Sleep domain ontology (SDO) contains standard terms representing sleep disorders, phenotypes, presentation, and medications as well as sleep procedures and devices, such as PSGs.[49] The concepts are stored using a formal logic language (such as the Web Ontology Language).[50]

Of specific interest to sleep medicine is the information available from the PSG, which contains physiologic and bioelectric signals, such as airflow, respiratory effort, EEG, electromyogram (EMG), electrooculogram (EOG), ECG, and oxygen saturation. This rich source of information has enormous potential for characterizing dynamic

---

Box 1
Establishing big data resources in sleep medicine

Creation of comprehensive archives of sleep study data

The collection of the data, sensors, scoring criteria, and recording should be standardized. However, technology is rapidly improving and evolving; avoiding getting locked down to an inferior option demands flexibility not generally considered in scientific investigations.

A structured format for health care data notes and documentation of laboratory results, imaging, genetic, and other studies will promote homogeneity of such databases.

A normalized vocabulary of sleep terms is required for cross-referencing and more valid comparisons.

The data must be stored on widely accessible platforms and retrievable through user-friendly interfaces to be of maximum value to the researchers.

Open access or nominal cost will help widespread utilization.

Frameworks need to be in place to better define data access from different sources to help share and communicate information.

Set up secure and largely automated data pathways to merge data from the EHR, sleep laboratory polysomnogram, therapeutic-device tracking systems, and data from wearables.

changes in neurophysiologic and cardiorespiratory parameters over a period of hours. Curation of data from multiple physiologic systems may allow a more improved characterization of sleep apnea–related stresses and may provide a rich source of physiologic data that describes multiple organ systems, including the interactions across those systems. Centralized and open-access libraries of well-defined PSGs from multiple studies and sites could enhance the objectives described in the preceding sections. Big data opportunities include those that ask questions, such as the following: Does a combination of signals, such as heart rate variability and EEG changes or flow pattern, define the outcomes better than traditionally used definitions of sleep apnea? Does a combination of signals provide a more reliable quantification of central versus obstructive origin of hypopneas? There are also opportunities to extract responses to PAP titration in systematic formats to identify subgroups of individuals, such as those with complex sleep apnea or with phenotypes, such as high loop gain.

There is a strong push, based on economic consideration among others, to increase the use of portable sleep testing devices. Portable systems frequently record a subset of signals used in PSG (frequently including airflow, respiratory effort, and oxygen saturation) and/or other signals, such a peripheral arterial tonometry. The use of portable systems can introduce a heterogeneous set of data and data collected in less controlled settings than laboratory-based assessments. Establishing standards for data quality for data derived from these portable systems is needed as those data are curated into larger data repositories.

A major concern when aggregating data relates to the comparability of the source or derived data. When harmonizing data from PSG or home sleep tests, it is important to recognize that the sensors used are variable in their material, mechanism of acquiring signal (pressure changes, temperature changes), validation process and reliability. Adherence to a common set of procedures for measurement and scoring improves the comparability of data from different sources and laboratories.[15,51] However, often data were collected when no or different data standards were in place, or were collected with equipment that uses different collection and processing algorithms despite meeting minimal published standards. In those cases when data were collected differently, it is critical that each measurement is defined with sufficient specificity to allow the user to make appropriate analysis decisions, and the provenance of those measurements is provided.

Data from sleep tests also provide opportunities to generate numerous quantitative measures that can be used in big data analyses to enhance discovery of new patterns and predictors of disease. The various signals on the polysomnogram provide risk signal analysis opportunities, at the level of individual signals, coupled signals (eg, cardiopulmonary coupling and cardiorespiratory synchronization), and network analysis of multiple signals. Traditionally, the 30-second sleep epoch is considered the basic unit of sleep data and is assigned a sleep stage irrespective of the significant heterogeneity that may exist in EEG within that epoch (alpha and delta rhythms, K-complexes, sleep spindles, and so forth). Information from each epoch is often collapsed and summarized rather than analyzed using quantitative methods that characterize all of the information within each epoch and the relationship of data in surrounding epochs. Spectral and nonlinear analyses of these variables (see the section later) might further enhance the information content of PSG data often presented in simpler summary or binary format. Linear methods like fast Fourier transform of EEG data reformat EEG into component frequency spectral patterns and can help elucidate pathologic EEG patterns and their relationship to outcomes.[18] These analyses need to appropriately consider challenges in analyzing such signals, such as assumptions of stationary and impact of artifact. The human brain is neither just deterministic nor fully stochastic, and its properties and signal generation are nonlinear.[52] Newer nonlinear machine learning techniques, such as support vector machines for EEG signal classification or multi-scale entropy analysis, can be informative regarding EEG changes in sleep apnea and provide more insight into diagnosis and correlates.[53] Unsupervised and supervised machine learning algorithms can be used to understand the pattern differences as well as correlate them with the presence or absence of significant disease.[54–56]

ELECTRONIC HEALTH RECORD DATA

EHRs constitute a valuable collection of patient health information and can be transformative for individual patients as well as public health. A systematic collection of patient records helps track care, assess quality and safety of care, and trigger alerts, warnings, and reminders. The Health Information Technology for Economic and Clinical Health Act was enacted as part of the American Recovery and Reinvestment Act of 2009 to promote the health information technology adoption, including certified EHR adoption, formation of patient registries, and achievement of meaningful use objectives. Use of electronic prescribing and cross-referencing with diagnoses can help keep track of the use of medications, such as hypnotics or stimulants, in patients with SDB and promote safety. Such data help understand which patients need these medications and how these medications impact diverse outcomes, such as sleep quality, quality of life, daytime sleepiness, traffic accidents, and so forth. Given the variation in SDB phenotypes across the population, the development of SDB registries could create resources to better understand the differences in risk factors, outcomes, and treatment responses across patients and, thus, inform more individualized screening, risk stratification, and treatment strategies. For example, registries can be used to identify patients with developmental disorders associated with OSA, patients with complex sleep apnea, patients with different levels of adherence, and patients with residual sleepiness despite sleep apnea treatment.[57] The American Academy of Sleep Medicine is in the process of publishing recommendations for sleep data to be included in the EHR that highlight end-to-end needs (from patient screening, diagnostic information, and population management) and are discussed (see Hwang D: Monitoring Progress and Adherence with Positive Airway Pressure Therapy for Obstructive Sleep Apnea: The Roles of Telemedicine and Mobile Health Applications, in this issue). The academy also reviewed and has recommended a list of recommended patient-reported surveys as well as data fields from sleep studies to be included in the EHR.

SLEEP MEDICINE BIG DATA RESOURCES

The NIH Big Data to Knowledge (BD2K) initiative was developed to support the development of state-of-the-art big data access and analysis methods. Its specific goals are to facilitate broad use of biomedical digital assets by making them discoverable, accessible, and citable; conduct research and develop the methods, software, and tools needed to analyze biomedical big data; enhance training in the development and use of methods and tools necessary for biomedical big data science and; support a data ecosystem that accelerates discovery as part of a digital enterprise. BD2K initiatives include the development of Centers of Excellence for big data computing, Data Discovery Coordination consortia, and big data courses and open educational resources. Although many of these initiatives are generic, at least one BD2K-funded project identifies sleep-related data as a use case for developing more

advanced approaches for data annotation and visualization. The White House Brain Research through Advancing Innovative Neurotechnologies initiative[58] defines a national research agenda to undercover mechanisms involved in neurologic diseases, such as Alzheimer disease, Parkinson disease, and depression, which are topics of relevance to the sleep medicine community.

In the past few years, there has been a concerted effort toward development of repositories of sleep data that are more comprehensive, easily accessible, and well annotated. These resources are aimed at satisfying the informatics and data resource needs in the sleep community for clinical and research purposes. Large diverse collections of data can help elucidate the effect of age, sex, and demographic variables on the clinical and polysomnographic presentation of sleep apnea, identify predictors that may optimize management of sleep apnea, and provide novel characterizations of the associations between SDB and adverse health effects, such as cardiovascular disorders. Such large data sources, especially when combined with genetic data, can help improve sleep apnea phenotyping and identify genetic fingerprints of sleep apnea and the associated consequences.

The NSRR, established through an NHLBI resource grant, supports the goals of the NIH BD2K initiative by providing researchers and trainees with access to deidentified well-annotated physiologic signals from curated sleep studies linked to data aggregated from large cohort studies and clinical trials.[59] Data sets that have been made available through this resource include sleep studies and covariate data from the Sleep Heart Health Study (SHHS), the Cleveland Family Study, the Heart Biomarker Evaluation in Apnea, the Study of Osteoporotic Fractures, the MrOS Sleep Study (Outcomes of Sleep Disorders in Older Men), the Cleveland Children's Sleep and Health Study, and the Childhood Adenotonsillectomy Trial. The NSRR implements a scalable architecture designed to accommodate expansion to incorporate data abstracted from ongoing cohort studies, planned clinical trials, and clinical resources, including current generation EHRs. Available covariate data includes demographic information, anthropometric parameters, physiologic measurements, medical history elements, and neurocognitive testing results. Files that can be downloaded from the NSRR include raw signal data, covariate data, and a suite of modifiable tools that can be used for signal processing and analysis. Measurements of key parameters from EEG, EOG, EMG, and ECG using open-source codes are available and ready for use by investigators for biostatistical analysis. A cross-dataset query interface has been developed to facilitate the collection, management, and sharing of data (**Fig. 1**).[60,61] A canonical data dictionary that maps study-specific data variables to a standardized set of variable definitions is used to standardize terminology across studies. This resource incorporates an expanding set of core terms drawn from a range of domains prioritized by their anticipated utility to facilitate intracohort exploratory data analysis and cross-cohort query generation. As each new dataset is added to the NSRR, an external data file is generated that maps core terms listed in the canonical data dictionary to corresponding study variables (**Fig. 2**). As each study variable is mapped, it is annotated with provenance attributes that specify the source of the data, the time point of collection, the method of collection, and the specifics of any equipment used to acquire the data.[62,63]

Social networking Web sites that contain personal, social, and occasionally medical information as well as Web sites designed specifically to disseminate medical information or allow active patient engagement are other valuable sources for big data.[3,64] The emerging big data models have allowed patients to generate and share their data rather than just relying on health care institutions for data accumulation. Crowdsourcing has recently been be used to help build prediction, detection, and therapeutic models. The current push is to allow an open-access model for such data, allowing democratization of the data.[43] Patients are now playing a role not only in generating the data but even analyzing and publishing it.[3,65] In this regard, a sleep apnea resource is the Sleep Apnea Patient Centered Outcomes Network and its public facing portal, MyApnea.Org.[3] This resource is a virtual network of patients, family members, clinicians, and researchers who interact through a forum and series of interactive tools, including tools for nominating and voting on research priorities and sleep apnea screening tools. In addition, patients provide self-reported survey information through a series of validated and new tools that assess a range of information from experience with diagnosis, treatments, symptoms, quality of life, and health conditions.[3] As of January 2016, more than 6300 individuals have joined the network, providing large amounts of data to help the community understand, from patients' perspectives, issues related to satisfaction with care, treatment outcomes, and comorbidities. Data are collected using a common data

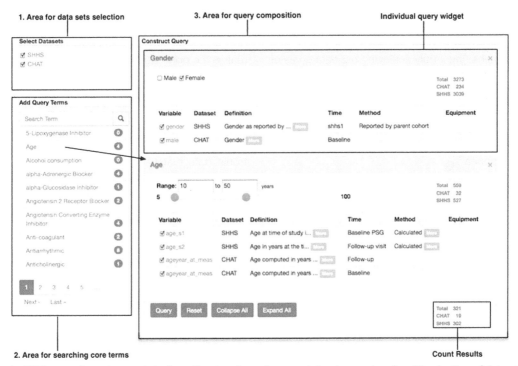

Fig. 1. NSRR cross-dataset query interface. Construction of a cross-dataset query involves (1) selection of datasets, (2) specification of core query terms, and (3) refinement of selectable parameters. A query returns counts of results annotated with attributes detailing the provenance of each included study variable. CHAT, Cross-country Historical Adoption of Technology (CHAT) dataset; SHHS, Sleep Heart Health Study.

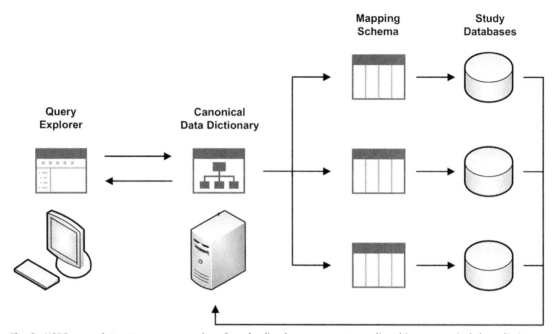

Fig. 2. NSRR cross-dataset query processing. Standardized core query terms listed in a canonical data dictionary are directly mapped to corresponding study variables in each dataset.

model, allowing integration with other national efforts. Such portals represent a significant evolution in patient engagement from being a mere participant to being the designers and drivers of the research. Over time, portals such as this may be enhanced by integrating information from wearables and PAP devices, EHR data, and biospecimens, thus, truly achieving big data goals of multidimensional data.

BioPortal provides a comprehensive repository of biomedical ontologies, including sleep ontologies.[66] PatientsLikeMe is another online data-sharing platform with millions of unique data points from patients with diverse disorders, including sleep apnea.[64]

LIMITATIONS AND CHALLENGES

Big data holds enormous promise but can be associated with significant challenges. Because data can come from several different sources, in different formats, with different annotations, harmonizing and standardizing can be a major undertaking. Although there exist some standards through the International Classification of Sleep Disorders and scoring manuals, and the NSRR has begun development of ontologies and metadata for sleep terms, there is not yet a nationally endorsed SDO. The disparate sources of sleep data across the medical system, from sleep laboratories to data collected by durable medical equipment companies to the use of wearable

medical devices and PAP machines, present special challenges for data capture and integration. New efforts by the American Academy of Sleep Medicine promise to begin the process for defining and prioritizing those items most relevant for sleep medicine. However, full participation by EHR vendors and health care systems will be required to realize the potential of these data. From the clinician's perspective, there will be further practical challenges. Data collection, access, and support need to improve both the efficiency and effectiveness of the clinical outcome to be of value and pragmatic. The role of regulatory and professional organizations in defining benchmarks for electronic data maintenance needs clarification and should enhance clinical care.

In establishing centralized data repositories or enhancing access to data, there are important privacy, security, and confidentiality concerns that need to be carefully and continuously addressed. However, there is also a need for the sleep medicine community to enhance its culture of collaboration whereby the value of sharing deidentified data and collaborative analysis is embraced. The public, funders, and industry all recognize that greater data sharing can improve transparency, enhance discovery, and accelerate dissemination of findings.[67] To achieve this goal, there is a need for the field to revisit traditional attitudes toward data ownership.

Volumes of data cannot compensate for poor-quality data, and defining and implementing data verification steps are critical. Big data can also lead to spurious outcomes if appropriate adjustment for multiple comparisons is not applied. Achieving a balance between heuristics and data-driven decision-making will need to be achieved until we have evidence of what is the most efficient and effective process to improve patient outcomes.[68,69]

Finally, big data can be extremely expensive to create and maintain. Collaborations between health care providers, information technologists, patient representatives, mathematicians, computer scientists, and statisticians, among others, as well as financial and regulatory support from federal, state, and private supporters will be required for maintenance and implementation of effective and viable clinical and research big data resources. It is imperative that the procurement, storage, and analytical methods be cost-efficient to be widely accepted and adopted and sustainable.

SUMMARY

Analysis of large-volume data holds the promise for improving the application of precision medicine to sleep, including improving the identification of patient subgroups who may specifically benefit from alternative therapies. Big data used within the health care system also promises to facilitate end-to-end screening, diagnosis and management of sleep disorders, improve the recognition of differences in presentation and susceptibility to sleep apnea, and lead to improved management and outcomes. To meet the vision of personalized, precision therapeutics and diagnostics and improving the efficiency and quality of sleep medicine will require ongoing efforts, investments, and some change in our current medical and research cultures. Expanding the EHR with well-defined sleep data and further development and growth of national research repositories and patient networks and registries are important strategies for achieving these goals. Any successful strategy will need to integrate patient-collected data through the rapidly evolving wearable device market.

REFERENCES

1. Tricoci P, Allen JM, Kramer JM, et al. Scientific evidence underlying the ACC/AHA clinical practice guidelines. JAMA 2009;301(8):831–41.
2. Prinz F, Schlange T, Asadullah K. Believe it or not: how much can we rely on published data on potential drug targets? Nat Rev Drug Discov 2011;10(9):712.
3. Available at: https://myapnea.org. Accessed December 25, 2015.
4. Mathur R, Douglas NJ. Family studies in patients with the sleep apnea-hypopnea syndrome. Ann Intern Med 1995;122(3):174–8.
5. Liu Y, Patel S, Nibbe R, et al. Systems biology analyses of gene expression and genome wide association study data in obstructive sleep apnea. Pac Symp Biocomput 2011;14–25.
6. Patel SR, Larkin EK, Redline S. Shared genetic basis for obstructive sleep apnea and adiposity measures. Int J Obes (Lond) 2008;32(5):795–800.
7. Larkin EK, Patel SR, Goodloe RJ, et al. A candidate gene study of obstructive sleep apnea in European Americans and African Americans. Am J Respir Crit Care Med 2010;182(7):947–53.
8. Patel SR, Goodloe R, De G, et al. Association of genetic loci with sleep apnea in European Americans and African-Americans: the candidate gene association resource (CARe). PLoS One 2012;7(11):e48836.
9. Gaziano JM, Concato J, Brophy M, et al. Million Veteran Program: a mega-biobank to study genetic influences on health and disease. J Clin Epidemiol 2015;70:214–23.
10. McCarty CA, Chisholm RL, Chute CG, et al. The eMERGE Network: a consortium of biorepositories linked to electronic medical records data for conducting genomic studies. BMC Med Genomics 2011;4(1):13.
11. Budhiraja R, Parthasarathy S, Quan SF. Endothelial dysfunction in obstructive sleep apnea. J Clin Sleep Med 2007;3(4):409–15.
12. Spira AP, Blackwell T, Stone KL, et al. Sleep-disordered breathing and cognition in older women. J Am Geriatr Soc 2008;56(1):45–50.
13. Gozal D, Capdevila OS, Kheirandish-Gozal L, et al. APOE epsilon 4 allele, cognitive dysfunction, and obstructive sleep apnea in children. Neurology 2007;69(3):243–9.
14. Nikodemova M, Finn L, Mignot E, et al. Association of sleep disordered breathing and cognitive deficit in APOE epsilon4 carriers. Sleep 2013;36(6):873–80.
15. Berry RB, Budhiraja R, Gottlieb DJ, et al. Rules for scoring respiratory events in sleep: update of the 2007 AASM manual for the scoring of sleep and associated events. Deliberations of the sleep apnea definitions task force of the American Academy of Sleep Medicine. J Clin Sleep Med 2012;8(5):597–619.
16. Budhiraja R, Goodwin JL, Parthasarathy S, et al. Comparison of nasal pressure transducer and thermistor for detection of respiratory events during polysomnography in children. Sleep 2005;28(9):1117–21.
17. Mokhlesi B, Finn LA, Hagen EW, et al. Obstructive sleep apnea during REM sleep and hypertension. Results of the Wisconsin sleep cohort. Am J Respir Crit Care Med 2014;190(10):1158–67.
18. Budhiraja R, Quan SF, Punjabi NM, et al. Power spectral analysis of the sleep electroencephalogram

in heartburn patients with or without gastroesophageal reflux disease: a feasibility study. J Clin Gastroenterol 2010;44(2):91–6.

19. Giffen CA, Carroll LE, Adams JT, et al. Providing contemporary access to historical biospecimen collections: development of the NHLBI Biologic Specimen and Data Repository Information Coordinating Center (BioLINCC). Biopreserv Biobank 2015; 13(4):271–9.

20. Goldberger AL, Amaral LA, Glass L, et al. PhysioBank, PhysioToolkit, and PhysioNet: components of a new research resource for complex physiologic signals. Circulation 2000;101(23):E215–20.

21. Moody GB, Mark RG, Goldberger AL. PhysioNet: physiologic signals, time series and related open source software for basic, clinical, and applied research. Conf Proc IEEE Eng Med Biol Soc 2011; 2011:8327–30.

22. Available at: http://www.sleepimage.com. Accessed January 19, 2016.

23. Available at: http://www.resmed.com/us/en/consumer/s-plus.html. Accessed January 19, 2016.

24. Johns MW. A new method for measuring daytime sleepiness: the Epworth sleepiness scale. Sleep 1991;14(6):540–5.

25. Johns MW. Sensitivity and specificity of the multiple sleep latency test (MSLT), the maintenance of wakefulness test and the Epworth sleepiness scale: failure of the MSLT as a gold standard. J Sleep Res 2000;9(1):5–11.

26. Budhiraja R, Parthasarathy S, Drake CL, et al. Early CPAP use identifies subsequent adherence to CPAP therapy. Sleep 2007;30(3):320–4.

27. Budhiraja R, Sharief I, Quan SF. Sleep disordered breathing and hypertension. J Clin Sleep Med 2005;1(4):401–4.

28. Dean DA, Wang R, Jacobs DR, et al. A systematic assessment of the association of polysomnographic indices with blood pressure: the multi-ethnic study of atherosclerosis (MESA). Sleep 2015;38(4):587–96.

29. Redline S, Sotres-Alvarez D, Loredo J, et al. Sleep-disordered breathing in Hispanic/Latino individuals of diverse backgrounds. The Hispanic Community Health Study/Study of Latinos. Am J Respir Crit Care Med 2014;189(3):335–44.

30. Budhiraja R, Quan SF. Sleep-disordered breathing and cardiovascular health. Curr Opin Pulm Med 2005;11(6):501–6.

31. Budhiraja R, Budhiraja P, Quan SF. Sleep-disordered breathing and cardiovascular disorders. Respir Care 2010;55(10):1322–32 [discussion: 1330–2].

32. Lin GM, Colangelo LA, Lloyd-Jones DM, et al. Association of sleep apnea and snoring with incident atrial fibrillation in the multi-ethnic study of atherosclerosis. Am J Epidemiol 2015;182(1):49–57.

33. Seicean S, Kirchner HL, Gottlieb DJ, et al. Sleep-disordered breathing and impaired glucose metabolism in normal-weight and overweight/obese individuals: the Sleep Heart Health Study. Diabetes Care 2008;31(5):1001–6.

34. Strand LB, Carnethon M, Biggs ML, et al. Sleep disturbances and glucose metabolism in older adults: the Cardiovascular Health Study. Diabetes Care 2015;38(11):2050–8.

35. Bakker JP, Weng J, Wang R, et al. Associations between obstructive sleep apnea, sleep duration, and abnormal fasting glucose. The multi-ethnic study of atherosclerosis. Am J Respir Crit Care Med 2015; 192(6):745–53.

36. Gelber RP, Redline S, Ross GW, et al. Associations of brain lesions at autopsy with polysomnography features before death. Neurology 2015;84(3): 296–303.

37. Molnar MZ, Mucsi I, Novak M, et al. Association of incident obstructive sleep apnoea with outcomes in a large cohort of US veterans. Thorax 2015;70(9):888–95.

38. Lutsey PL, McClelland RL, Duprez D, et al. Objectively measured sleep characteristics and prevalence of coronary artery calcification: the Multi-Ethnic Study of Atherosclerosis Sleep study. Thorax 2015;70(9): 880–7.

39. Priou P, Le Vaillant M, Meslier N, et al. Cumulative association of obstructive sleep apnea severity and short sleep duration with the risk for hypertension. PLoS One 2014;9(12):e115666.

40. Phillips B, Shafazand S. CPAP and hypertension in nonsleepy patients. J Clin Sleep Med 2013;9(2): 181–2.

41. Shah N, Allison M, Teng Y, et al. Sleep apnea is independently associated with peripheral arterial disease in the Hispanic Community Health Study/Study of Latinos. Arterioscler Thromb Vasc Biol 2015;35(3):710–5.

42. Roca GQ, Redline S, Claggett B, et al. Sex-specific association of sleep apnea severity with subclinical myocardial injury, ventricular hypertrophy, and heart failure risk in a community-dwelling cohort: the atherosclerosis risk in communities-sleep heart health study. Circulation 2015; 132(14):1329–37.

43. Küffner R, Zach N, Norel R, et al. Crowdsourced analysis of clinical trial data to predict amyotrophic lateral sclerosis progression. Nat Biotechnol 2015; 33(1):51–7.

44. Shipley JE, Schteingart DE, Tandon R, et al. Sleep architecture and sleep apnea in patients with Cushing's disease. Sleep 1992;15(6):514–8.

45. Minic M, Granton JT, Ryan CM. Sleep disordered breathing in group 1 pulmonary arterial hypertension. J Clin Sleep Med 2014;10(3):277–83.

46. Mermigkis C, Stagaki E, Tryfon S, et al. How common is sleep-disordered breathing in patients with idiopathic pulmonary fibrosis? Sleep Breath 2010; 14(4):387–90.

47. Ezzat H, Mohab A. Prevalence of sleep disorders among ESRD patients. Ren Fail 2015;37(6):1013–9.

48. Maris M, Verhulst S, Wojciechowski M, et al. Prevalence of obstructive sleep apnea in children with down syndrome. Sleep 2015. [Epub ahead of print].

49. Arabandi S, Ogbuji C, Redline S, et al. Developing a sleep domain ontology (Abstract). In: Proceedings of the 2010 AMIA Clinical Research Informatics Summit. San Fransisco, CA, March 12–13, 2010.

50. Hitzler P, Krötzsch M, Parsia B, et al. OWL 2 web ontology language primer. World Wide Web Consortium (W3C) recommendation. 2009.

51. Redline S, Budhiraja R, Kapur V, et al. The scoring of respiratory events in sleep: reliability and validity. J Clin Sleep Med 2007;3(2):169–200.

52. Klonowski W. Everything you wanted to ask about EEG but were afraid to get the right answer. Nonlinear Biomed Phys 2009;3(1):2.

53. Khandoker AH, Palaniswami M, Karmakar CK. Support vector machines for automated recognition of obstructive sleep apnea syndrome from ECG recordings. IEEE Trans Inf Technol Biomed 2009; 13(1):37–48.

54. Gentleman R, Carey V. Unsupervised machine learning. In: Bioconductor case studies. Springer; 2008. p. 137–57.

55. Kotsiantis SB, Zaharakis I, Pintelas P. Supervised machine learning: a review of classification techniques. 2007.

56. Alpaydin E. Introduction to machine learning. MIT press; 2014.

57. Strollo PJ Jr, Badr MS, Coppola MP, et al. The future of sleep medicine. Sleep 2011;34(12):1613.

58. Bargmann CI, Newsome WT. The brain research through advancing innovative neurotechnologies (BRAIN) initiative and neurology. JAMA Neurol 2014;71(6):675–6.

59. Available at: https://sleepdata.org/. Accessed December 25, 2015.

60. Available at: http://www.nih.gov/news/health/jan2009/ncrr-26.htm. Accessed March 8, 2016.

61. Physio-MIMI. Available at: https://sleepdata.org/tools/physiomimi, Accessed December 25, 2015.

62. Zhang GQ, Siegler T, Saxman P, et al. VISAGE: a query interface for clinical research. In: Proceedings of the 2010 AMIA Clinical Research Informatics Summit. San Francisco, CA, March 12–13, 2010. p. 76–80.

63. Mueller R, Sahoo S, Dong X, et al. Mapping multi-institution data sources to domain ontology for data federation: the Physio-MIMI approach. American Medical Informatics Association Clinical Research Informatics Summit (CRI), 2011.

64. Wicks P, Massagli M, Frost J, et al. Sharing health data for better outcomes on PatientsLikeMe. J Med Internet Res 2010;12(2):e19.

65. Wicks P, Vaughan TE, Massagli MP, et al. Accelerated clinical discovery using self-reported patient data collected online and a patient-matching algorithm. Nat Biotechnol 2011;29(5):411–4.

66. Musen MA, Musen M, Shah NH, et al. BioPortal: ontologies and data resources with the click of a mouse. AMIA Annu Symp Proc 2008;6:1223–4.

67. Drazen JM. Sharing individual patient data from clinical trials. N Engl J Med 2015;372(3):201–2.

68. Cresswell K, Majeed A, Bates DW, et al. Computerised decision support systems for healthcare professionals: an interpretative review. Inform Prim Care 2012;20(2):115–28.

69. Marewski JN, Gigerenzer G. Heuristic decision making in medicine. Dialogues Clin Neurosci 2012;14(1): 77–89.

Advances and New Approaches to Managing Sleep-Disordered Breathing Related to Chronic Pulmonary Disease

Ronaldo A. Sevilla Berrios, MD[a,1], Peter C. Gay, MD[b,*]

KEYWORDS

- Sleep-disorder breathing • Chronic pulmonary disease • Noninvasive ventilation

KEY POINTS

In aggregate, it can be concluded that the evidence so far indicates subgroups that may benefit from home noninvasive ventilation (NIV):

- The patient with elevated $Paco_2$ (baseline >52 mm Hg) in chronic stable state.
- Possibly those hypercapnic patients with chronic obstructive pulmonary disease (COPD) admitted to the hospital with acute or chronic respiratory failure to avoid hospital readmissions.
- The routine use of higher inflation pressure and higher backup rate could potentially leverage the efficacy of chronic nocturnal noninvasive ventilation to the benefit of patients with severe COPD.

INTRODUCTION

Chronic obstructive pulmonary disease (COPD) is a very common disease affecting about 20 million US adults as of 2011.[1] It is also one of the most frequent causes of mortality in Americans. It was recognized as the third leading cause of death in the United States in 2009 with about 130,000 reported deaths related to this condition.[1,2] Furthermore, it represents a high cost to the US health care system, with nearly $50 billion per year spent on COPD management and hospital readmissions due to COPD exacerbations, making it imperative to develop therapies and strategies that can decrease this cost.

On the other hand, sleep-disordered breathing (SDB) problems are frequent and poorly characterized for patients with COPD. After daytime dyspnea and fatigue, sleep disturbances, including snoring, sleep apnea syndromes, and nocturnal hypoventilation, is considered the third most common complaint in patients with COPD.[3] The relationship between the presence of SDB and more severe clinically relevant outcomes in this population, including COPD exacerbation requiring emergency department visits, hospitalization, and all-cause mortality, has been well described.[4]

Both the well-known success of noninvasive ventilation (NIV) in the acute COPD exacerbation in the hospital setting[5] and that fact that NIV is the cornerstone of chronic therapy for SDBs have urged the attention of the medical community to determine the impact of NIV on chronic COPD management with and without coexisting SDBs. Over the past 3 decades, conflicting results of

[a] Critical Care Medicine, University of Pittsburg Medical Center at Hamot, Erie, PA 15650, USA; [b] Pulmonary, Critical Care and Sleep Medicine, Mayo Clinic, 200 1st Street Southwest, Rochester, MN 55905, USA
[1] Present address: 201 State Street, Erie, PA 16550.
* Corresponding author.
E-mail address: pgay@mayo.edu

Sleep Med Clin 11 (2016) 257–264
http://dx.doi.org/10.1016/j.jsmc.2016.01.002
1556-407X/16/$ – see front matter © 2016 Elsevier Inc. All rights reserved

studies have yielded inconclusive data whether regular use of nocturnal NIV to treat chronic respiratory failure in patients with COPD is cost-effective or not. More recently, technological advances in the use, functionality, and tolerability of NIV coupled with increased clinical expertise of sleep physicians have opened the door to a better understanding of the role for NIV as a part of the treatment arsenal for severe COPD and chronic respiratory failure. Newer high-flow humidified oxygen delivery systems and the possibility of respiratory stimulant medications are attempting to revolutionize this field; however, their roles are not fully understood yet.

SLEEP PHYSIOLOGY, CHRONIC OBSTRUCTIVE PULMONARY DISEASE, AND SLEEP-DISORDERED BREATHING

Physiologic changes in the chemoreceptors' sensitivity to CO_2 and alterations in $Paco_2$ occur in healthy individuals routinely during normal sleep. Changes in minute ventilation with a subsequent decrease in oxygenation can be seen in deeper stages of sleep and are maximum during rapid eye movement sleep.[6] These changes are accentuated in patients with COPD, leading to a further decrease in receptors' chemosensitivity; thus, hypercapnia and hypoxemia are greater in this patient population.[7,8]

The presence of obstructive sleep apnea (OSA) or obesity hypoventilation syndrome in patients with COPD moves the ventilatory responsiveness to the flatter part of their respective hypercapnic and hypoxic response curves. As a result, dulling of the ventilatory responsiveness can induce more pronounced hypercapnia and/or hypoxia in these patients.[9] Screening of patients with severe COPD with oximetry suggests that 10% to 20% of patients may have some type of additional SDB, making this problem extremely relevant.[10,11]

REVIEW OF RECENT DATA REGARDING NOCTURNAL NONINVASIVE VENTILATION ON PATIENTS WITH CHRONIC OBSTRUCTIVE PULMONARY DISEASE

Most observational studies showed a marked decrease in long-term survival rates in patients with COPD with concomitant chronic respiratory failure evidenced by chronic hypercapnia when compared with normocapnic patients,[12] although this also has some level of controversy.[13,14] In the early 2000s, studies investigated if normalization of hypercapnia using NIV could have an impact on the prognosis of patients with COPD with chronic respiratory failure. Initial data suggested

that routine NIV usage aimed to normalize the arterial partial pressure of carbon dioxide ($Paco_2$) on patients with COPD in the home setting did not have an impact on hospitalization or mortality but worsened quality of life (QOL).[15] In 2009, McEvoy and colleagues[16] conducted a large randomized controlled trial in Australia including 144 patients with COPD on long-term oxygen therapy and $Paco_2$ greater than 46 mm Hg. They tested the usage of NIV for 3 hours targeted to a pressure support (PS) of 10 cm H_2O versus standard therapy that showed minimal survival benefit with worsening general and mental health.[16] A report based on a meta-analysis of 7 studies that included 245 patients from the Cochrane Collaboration in 2013 concluded that NIV has "no clinically or statistically significant effect on gas exchange, exercise tolerance, quality of life (QOL), lung function, respiratory muscle strength or sleep efficiency and should only be use in the connection of a clinical trial."[17]

Recently, Köhnlein and colleagues[18] randomized 195 patients from 36 respiratory units in Germany and Austria to receive either standard therapy or standard therapy plus NIV and followed these patients for a minimum of 1 year. They reported an absolute mortality risk reduction of 21% (33% vs 12%, P<.01) (**Fig. 1**) with remarkable tolerability and minimal side effects (facial rash in 14% of patients in the intervention group that resolved after interface exchange) despite the use of high pressures and a backup rate (described in later discussion). Patients included had stage IV COPD with resting average $Paco_2$ of 51.9 mm Hg or higher and pH >7.35. All the clinical

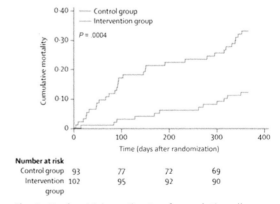

Fig. 1. Kaplan-Meier estimate of cumulative all-cause mortality during the first year after randomization (primary outcome). (*From* Köhnlein T, Windisch W, Köhler D, et al. Non-invasive positive pressure ventilation for the treatment of severe stable chronic obstructive pulmonary disease: a prospective, multi-centre, randomised, controlled clinical trial. Lancet Respir Med 2014;2(9):703; with permission.)

characteristics of the 2 groups were comparable, and the follow-up was adequate for clinical extrapolation. This study differed from other studies, in that patients in this trial were targeted to a reduction of $Paco_2$ by at least 20% or a $Paco_2$ lower than 48.1 instead of just seeking PS level target as in most other studies. Also, the investigators preset a higher backup rate (18–22 breaths per minute) in order to assure a bigger minute ventilation. Also, it is noteworthy that patients used the device an average of 5.6 hours per night, which was significantly higher than previous studies, wherein average usage was about 3 hours per night.

This data impacted the clinical community because it differed significantly with previous published studies. This difference may be accounted for by the NIV settings (higher inflation pressures and higher backup rate) that lead to greater normalization of $Paco_2$. Although critics have claimed some level of bias in this study, including that it was an unblinded study and possibly led to differences in treatment from the medical personal. There was also a high level of selectivity (about 1 patient per center per year and it took 7 years to enroll all the patients). Finally, the opportunity for NIV treatment was restrictive in the control arm until $Paco_2$ was greater than 75 mm Hg (which is above the usual recommendation), which could have led to overexpression of the differences from other studies as described.

Struik and colleagues[19] also attempted to evaluate further this therapeutic NIV strategy. They assessed the role of NIV on preventing hospital readmission on patients with COPD that required NIV during the initial hospitalization for acute COPD exacerbation and acute hypercapnic respiratory failure. They evaluated 201 patients with global obstructive lung disease (GOLD) stage 3 or 4 who had a minimal $Paco_2$ level of 55 mm Hg. They used similar high-pressure settings with a backup rate of 16/min, similar to Köhnlein and colleagues,[18] and compliance averaged 6.3 hours per night. However, they failed to show any significant reduction on hospital readmission, mortality, or COPD exacerbation rates after 1 year of therapy. The QOL indices trended toward improvement in health-related issues. It is possible that the Struik study population was in fact different than Köhnlein and colleagues', because in the Struik study their $Paco_2$ levels may have still been recovering from elevations due to their recent COPD exacerbation as opposed to a chronic severe stable state. This finding can become evident when the control group was analyzed, wherein they also had "spontaneous" resolution/normalization of their $Paco_2$ levels despite not been treated with NIV therapy. Also,

other factors leading to the initial hospitalization were not well delineated, such as medical therapy compliance or development new comorbidities such as sleep-disordered breathing.

Another study that is worth discussing (**Fig. 2**) was conducted by Galli and colleagues.[20] This group retrospectively observed patients admitted to their medical center for COPD due to an acute hypercapnic exacerbation and treated with NIV acutely during that hospitalization. They followed those that used NIV at home and compared them with those that did not. Although the group with home NIV were sicker (lower vital capacity) and had higher prevalence of OSA and obesity hypoventilation syndrome, they also had significantly higher event-free survival compared with the control group with a reduction in hospital readmission (40% vs 75%, $P<.01$) at 6-month follow up.

Again, it is difficult to draw a definitive conclusion with the data available as these conflicting results are hard to interpret. However, it is relevant that the subgroup of patients that had showed greater benefit is the one that had the combination of OSA and COPD also known as the "overlap syndrome."[21]

In aggregate, it can be concluded that the evidence so far identifies subgroups that may benefit from home NIV: (1) patients with elevated baseline in chronic stable state greater than 52 mm Hg[18,22]; (2) possibly on those hypercapnic patients with COPD admitted to the hospital with acute or chronic respiratory failure[20,23]; (3) the continuous nocturnal use of higher inflation pressure and higher backup rate could potentially leverage the efficacy of chronic nocturnal NIV in patients with

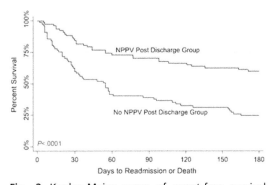

Fig. 2. Kaplan-Meier curve of event-free survival comparing patients who used noninvasive positive pressure ventilation (NPPV) after discharge versus patients who did not use NPPV after discharge. (*From* Galli JA, Krahnke JS, Mamary AJ, et al. Home non-invasive ventilation use following acute hypercapnic respiratory failure in COPD. Respir Med 2014;108(5):726; with permission.)

severe COPD[18]; (4) patients with overlap syndrome[20,24] (**Table 1**).

VOLUME TARGET NONINVASIVE VENTILATION FOR HYPERCAPNIA IN CHRONIC RESPIRATORY FAILURE

Customarily, home NIV is achieved by first setting a predetermined expiratory positive airway pressure (EPAP) and inspiratory positive airway pressure (IPAP) whereby the volume delivered is variable and dependent of the pressure difference between IPAP and EPAP (the PS) and the anatomic characteristics of the patients airway and respiratory system compliance.[25] In order to obtain a more reliable delivery of a set tidal volume and minute ventilation, a new strategy was developed based on volume-assured PS ventilation on intubated patients for acute respiratory failure. In the NIV modality called volume-targeted bilevel positive airway pressure (VT-BPAP), a set EPAP pressure and a varying IPAP (range from a set minimum to a maximum IPAP) led to a variable PS. The machine then self-adjusts the IPAP in the preset range to increase or decrease the PS in order to deliver a targeted tidal volume.[26,27]

The theoretic value of VT-BPAP over standard pressure-targeted NIV strategies has never been documented. Tuggey and Elliott[28] enrolled 13 patients with chronic respiratory failure secondary to chest wall abnormalities in a crossover randomized blind study comparing pressure versus volume-target mode of NIV. They could not find significant differences in sleep quality, daytime arterial blood gas tensions, lung mechanics, ventilatory drive, health status, or daytime functioning. As such, they concluded that these 2 modes of NIV were equivalent in this patient population. Windisch and colleagues[29] tested these 2 modalities in a prospective randomized crossover trial in 15 patients with chronic respiratory failure (9 of them due to COPD and 6 of them for other various causes). Unfortunately, only two-thirds of the study population completed the study, making their results unclear and limited. With the available patients, they did not find evidence of significant clinical or polysomnographic differences. They also concluded that these 2 strategies were therefore equivalent.

Finally, another somewhat similar strategy available is intelligent volume-assured pressure support (iVAPS). It differed from traditional VT-BPAP in that the goal of ventilation is based on minute ventilation as opposed to tidal volume. It is achieved through an automatic increase in backup rate and continuously monitored and reassessed average delivered ventilation.[30] Kelly and colleagues[31] randomized iVAPs versus pressure target BPAP strategy in patients with chronic respiratory failure. Although they confirmed lower IPAPmax in the iVAPS group, they did not find a difference on spirometry, respiratory muscle strength, sleep quality, number of arousals, or oxygen desaturation indexes. As a final point, they concluded that both therapies were equivalent in effectiveness. Currently, a Canadian group is recruiting patients with chronic respiratory failure secondary to amyotrophic lateral sclerosis to a prospective randomized trial where iVAPS will be compared with traditional pressure target BPAP strategy.[32] More information of long-term outcomes regarding the effectiveness of this therapy is needed.

NONINVASIVE VENTILATION REIMBURSEMENT ISSUES

Currently in the United States, most patients rely on insurance to obtain home NIV devices, also termed as respiratory assistance devices (RADs) by the Centers for Medicare and Medicaid (CMS). Otherwise, this machine might have a prohibitive personal cost when the expense of the machine itself and the long-term cost of frequently renewing supplies such as interface, tubing, and filters are factored in. However, current insurance regulations primarily based on CMS reimbursement criteria are exceedingly strict with specific coverage criteria that are often difficult to understand and meet. For the patient to obtain such a device, the sleep medicine specialists must document the precise expected language in order to fulfill those criteria. In overlap syndrome patients, they can often easily obtain CPAP equipment due to their documented OSA diagnosis; however, in the United States, they must fail this therapy to transition to NIV therapy and then only in the spontaneous rate mode without a backup rate. For this, there has to be documentation of "CPAP was tried and proven ineffective." Because this term of "ineffectiveness" is nonspecific, it can be used in multiple circumstances, including (1) patient intolerance to therapy, (2) poor adherence to therapy, (3) lack of achievement of therapeutic goals, but the documentation is still challenging.

Last, in order to get an NIV with a backup rate, it has to be proven that hypercapnia is worsening or that there are continued desaturations uncontrolled on NIV spontaneous mode and that it was improved or resolved by adding a backup rate. When all these criteria are met, then the patient can potentially receive their NIV with a backup rate. In the face of imprecise outcome data, it is easy to see that this approach would most likely

Table 1
Summary of recent studies evaluating efficacy of noninvasive ventilation therapy of patients with chronic obstructive pulmonary disease with chronic respiratory failure

Author	Population	Methodology	Intervention	Results
McEvoy et al,[16] 2009	144 patients with COPD on long-term oxygen therapy and $Paco_2$ >46 mm Hg	Randomized controlled trial	NIV for 3 h target to a PS of 10 cm H_2O vs standard therapy	Minimal survival benefit with worsening general and mental health
Struik et al,[17] 2013; Struik et al,[19] 2014	201 patients with GOLD stage 3 or 4 who had at least a $Paco_2$ level elevated to 55 mm Hg	Randomized controlled trial	High-inflation pressure, high backup rate of 16 breaths/min, and compliance average of 6.3 h per night vs standard therapy	It did not show any significant reduction on hospital readmission, mortality, COPD exacerbation after 1 y of therapy. It trended to improve QOL
Köhnlein et al,[18] 2014	195 patients from 36 respiratory units in Germany and Austria stage IV COPD with resting $Paco_2$ ≥51.9 mm Hg and pH >7.35	Randomized controlled trial	Standard therapy vs NIV with backup rate 18–22 bpm with goal to decrease $Paco_2$ >20% or >48 mm Hg for about 1 y and average usage was 5.6 h per night	Absolute mortality risk reduction of 21%
Galli et al,[20] 2014	166 patients hospitalized for COPD exacerbation that also required NIV for acute hypercapnic respiratory failure	Retrospective observational	No intervention. Patients were divided into 2 groups: those that NIV was prescribed at hospitalization discharge and used it vs those that were treated with standard medical therapy	Patients had a higher event-free survival compared with the control group with a reduction in hospital readmission (40% vs 75%, $P<.01$) at 6 mo

delay the initiation of a potentially quality-improving/survival-increasing therapy.

RECOMMENDATION FOR REVISION OF CURRENT GUIDELINE OF CHRONIC OBSTRUCTIVE PULMONARY DISEASE TREATMENT WITH NONINVASIVE VENTILATION DEVICES

The authors think that current guidelines of coverage for NIV on patients with COPD and SDB delay therapy initiation and may obstruct potential benefit especially for the more severe patients. With the current regulations, before NIV therapy, initiation with a backup rate on patients with severe COPD, the spontaneous mode must be demonstrated as ineffective in some cases for up to 90 days before moving on to other therapy. Considering the Galli study,[20] the patients with the overlap syndrome are the ones more likely to benefit from NIV therapy with a backup rate as is done routinely in Europe.

Considering the above, the authors recommend the initiation of NIV therapy with a backup rate for patients with severe COPD (GOLD stage 3 or 4 airway obstruction), with an arterial blood gas collected while awake and breathing of the usual Fio_2, showing that $Paco_2$ is greater than or equal to 52 mm Hg (**Fig. 3**). Based on the current evidence from the Köhnlein and colleagues[18] and Galli and colleagues[20] studies reviewed earlier, patients with severe COPD and chronic respiratory failure evidenced by CO_2 retention are the patients more likely to benefit from high-inflation pressure and high backup rates.

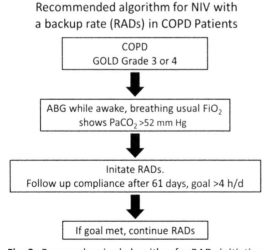

Recommended algorithm for NIV with a backup rate (RADs) in COPD Patients

Fig. 3. Proposed revised algorithm for RADs initiation on patients with COPD. ABG, arterial blood gas.

HIGH-FLOW HUMIDIFIED OXYGEN DELIVERY DEVICES

High-flow oxygen devices are capable of delivering up to 60 L/min of heated and humidified oxygen usually through a large-bore nasal cannula. This concept has been most well studied in pediatric patients and in critically ill adults with hypoxemic respiratory failure without hypercapnia. Kubicka and colleagues[33] evaluated the pressure generated by heated humidified high-flow (HHHF) nasal oxygen in infants and measured pressure as high as 4.5 cm H_2O with flow rates of 8 L/min. Other researchers have replicated this finding in healthy adults using HHHF and breathing with their mouth closed.[34] It has been postulated that HHHF can be used in patients with overlap syndrome without significant hypercapnia that are poorly tolerant to traditional CPAP therapy. To date, there are no studies that have evaluated this hypothesis, so there is a need for further research in this field.

RESPIRATORY STIMULANTS DRUGS FOR CHRONIC RESPIRATORY FAILURE

Although this approach is not well validated, recently, a growing body of literature has tried to give direction in whether pharmacologic approaches are valid options for patients with chronic respiratory failure. Parnell and colleagues[35] reported their experience treating 6 patients with acute or chronic respiratory failure that refused NIV therapy, by using Modafinil with the objective to stimulate their respiratory drive and resolve CO_2 retention. Patients were followed up for about 10 days in hospital with clear improvement in their hypercapnia. In addition, patients remained on Modafinil off-label usage with a decrease in hospital readmission rates for up to 1 year of follow-up. The reason for this improvement is unclear because there were no significant changes on pulmonary function testing; it was hypothesized to be related to the direct stimulation of the respiratory center in the central nervous system.

Yokoba and colleagues[36] evaluated the effect of aminophylline, previously used primarily as a bronchodilator that works mechanistically through nonselective phosphodiesterase inhibition and nonselective adenosine receptor antagonism, with potential central nervous system stimulant properties. Seven healthy volunteers with induced hypercapnia were evaluated before and after treatment with this medication. They showed an increase in minute ventilation and increased electromyogram activity of both inspiratory and expiratory muscles, suggesting a potential clinical utility in patients with chronic respiratory failure. To this date, this hypothesis is yet to be been tested.

Anttalainen and colleagues[37] explored the effects of medroxyprogesterone (MPG) in postmenopausal patients with SDB. They followed 34 patients for more than 6 weeks and found a significant decrease in $Paco_2$ in the treatment group. This effect was present over and above the effect of CPAP therapy. They concluded that MPG does have stimulant effects on the respiratory center; however, it was not sufficient to correct OSA alone. They postulate that it could be used in conjunction with CPAP therapy on patients with increased $Paco_2$ chronically.

Currently, a reliable pharmacologic therapy targeting hypercapnia in COPD and SDB patients is not yet proven. Further research is needed.

SUMMARY

In conclusion, the evidence regarding NIV on COPD showed some inconsistent results, but the latest studies using newer machines and improved algorithms and technology seem to show benefit on those patients with COPD and chronic respiratory failure as evidenced by higher levels of $Paco_2$ (52 mm Hg or greater). Benefit may be greatest in those patients with severe COPD GOLD stage 3 or 4 or the patient with overlap syndrome (coexisting OSA and COPD) especially when higher inflation pressures and higher backup rates were used. As such, the authors are not aware of evidence that supports the current approach for coverage qualification in the American health system and recommend change in RAD regulations. They propose early initiation of NIV with high backup rate on those patients that fulfill the description stated earlier.

Even though other ventilation strategies including VT-BPAP and iVAPs are available, they have not been shown to have a significant outcome benefit over the current pressure targeted ventilation modes, and they may be significantly more costly. Neither HHHF oxygen nor possible pharmacologic therapies are well studied as yet so they should not be used in routine clinical practice. Combination therapies might offer a further new horizon to explore for future benefit to patients with chronic respiratory failure.

REFERENCES

1. Ford ES, Croft JB, Mannino DM, et al. COPD surveillance—United States, 1999-2011. Chest 2013; 144(1):284–305.
2. Mannino DM, Doherty DE, Buist AS. Global Initiative on Obstructive Lung Disease (GOLD) classification of lung disease and mortality: findings from the Atherosclerosis Risk In Communities (ARIC) study. Respir Med 2006;100(1):115–22.
3. Kinsman R, Yaroush R, Fernandez E, et al. Symptoms and experiences in chronic bronchitis and emphysema. Chest 1983;83(5):755–61.
4. Omachi TA, Blanc PD, Claman DM, et al. Disturbed sleep among COPD patients is longitudinally associated with mortality and adverse COPD outcomes. Sleep Med 2012;13(5):476–83.
5. Plant P, Owen J, Elliott M. Early use of non-invasive ventilation for acute exacerbations of chronic obstructive pulmonary disease on general respiratory wards: a multicentre randomised controlled trial. Lancet 2000;355(9219):1931–5.
6. Phillipson EA. Control of breathing during sleep 1, 2. Am Rev Respir Dis 1978;118(5):909–39.
7. O'Donoghue FJ, Catcheside PG, Ellis E, et al. Sleep hypoventilation in hypercapnic chronic obstructive pulmonary disease: prevalence and associated factors. Eur Respir J 2003;21(6):977–84.
8. Gay PC. Chronic obstructive pulmonary disease and sleep. Respir Care 2004;49(1):39–52.
9. Budhiraja R, Siddiqi TA, Quan SF. Sleep disorders in chronic obstructive pulmonary disease: etiology, impact, and management. J Clin Sleep Med 2014; 11(3):259–70.
10. Brander P, Kuitunen T, Salmi T, et al. Nocturnal oxygen saturation in advanced chronic obstructive pulmonary disease after a moderate dose of ethanol. Eur Respir J 1992;5(3):308–12.
11. Kutty K. Sleep and chronic obstructive pulmonary disease. Curr Opin Pulm Med 2004;10(2):104–12.
12. Foucher P, Baudouin N, Merati M, et al. Relative survival analysis of 252 patients with COPD receiving long-term oxygen therapy. Chest 1998;113(6):1580–7.
13. Barach A. The adaptive function of hypercapnia. Chronic obstructive pulmonary disease. New York: Dekker; 1978.
14. Petty TL. CO2 can be good for you! Chest 2006; 129(2):494–5.
15. Rossi A. Noninvasive ventilation has not been shown to be ineffective in stable COPD. Am J Respir Crit Care Med 2000;161(3):688–9.
16. McEvoy RD, Pierce RJ, Hillman D, et al. Nocturnal non-invasive nasal ventilation in stable hypercapnic COPD: a randomised controlled trial. Thorax 2009; 64(7):561–6.
17. Struik FM, Lacasse Y, Goldstein R, et al. Nocturnal non-invasive positive pressure ventilation for stable chronic obstructive pulmonary disease. Cochrane Database Syst Rev 2013;(6):CD002878.
18. Köhnlein T, Windisch W, Köhler D, et al. Non-invasive positive pressure ventilation for the treatment of severe stable chronic obstructive pulmonary disease: a prospective, multicentre, randomised, controlled clinical trial. Lancet Respir Med 2014;2(9):698–705.

19. Struik F, Sprooten R, Kerstjens H, et al. Nocturnal non-invasive ventilation in COPD patients with prolonged hypercapnia after ventilatory support for acute respiratory failure: a randomised, controlled, parallel-group study. Thorax 2014;69(9):826–34.

20. Galli JA, Krahnke JS, Mamary AJ, et al. Home non-invasive ventilation use following acute hypercapnic respiratory failure in COPD. Respir Med 2014; 108(5):722–8.

21. Masa JF, Corral J, Alonso ML, et al. Efficacy of different treatment alternatives for obesity hypoventilation syndrome. Pickwick study. Am J Respir Crit Care Med 2015;192(1):86–95.

22. Meecham Jones DJ, Paul EA, Jones PW, et al. Nasal pressure support ventilation plus oxygen compared with oxygen therapy alone in hypercapnic COPD. Am J Respir Crit Care Med 1995;152(2):538–44.

23. Casanova C, Celli BR, Tost L, et al. Long-term controlled trial of nocturnal nasal positive pressure ventilation in patients with severe COPD. Chest 2000;118(6):1582–90.

24. Windisch W, Storre JH, Kohnlein T. Nocturnal non-invasive positive pressure ventilation for COPD. Expert Rev Respir Med 2015;9(3):295–308.

25. Sanders MH, Moore SE. Inspiratory and expiratory partitioning of airway resistance during sleep in patients with sleep apnea 1, 2. Am Rev Respir Dis 1983;127(5):554–8.

26. Gentina T, Fortin F, Douay B, et al. Auto bi-level with pressure relief during exhalation as a rescue therapy for optimally treated obstructive sleep apnoea patients with poor compliance to continuous positive airways pressure therapy—a pilot study. Sleep Breath 2011;15(1):21–7.

27. Storre JH, Seuthe B, Fiechter R, et al. Average volume-assured pressure support in obesity hypoventilation: a randomized crossover trial. Chest 2006;130(3):815–21.

28. Tuggey JM, Elliott MW. Randomised crossover study of pressure and volume non-invasive ventilation in chest wall deformity. Thorax 2005;60(10):859–64.

29. Windisch W, Storre JH, Sorichter S, et al. Comparison of volume-and pressure-limited NPPV at night: a prospective randomized cross-over trial. Respir Med 2005;99(1):52–9.

30. Thomas R. Positive pressure titration. Atlas of Sleep Medicine. Philadelphia: Elsevier Saunders; 2013. p. 300.

31. Kelly JL, Jaye J, Pickersgill RE, et al. Randomized trial of 'intelligent' autotitrating ventilation versus standard pressure support non-invasive ventilation: impact on adherence and physiological outcomes. Respirology 2014;19(4):596–603.

32. Kaminska M. Non-invasive ventilation in amyotrophic lateral sclerosis (ALS) using the iVAPS mode. Pulmonary Medicine and Rehab 2015;7(7):677–84.

33. Kubicka ZJ, Limauro J, Darnall RA. Heated, humidified high-flow nasal cannula therapy: yet another way to deliver continuous positive airway pressure? Pediatrics 2008;121(1):82–8.

34. Groves N, Tobin A. High flow nasal oxygen generates positive airway pressure in adult volunteers. Aust Crit Care 2007;20(4):126–31.

35. Parnell H, Quirke G, Farmer S, et al. The successful treatment of hypercapnic respiratory failure with oral modafinil. Int J Chron Obstruct Pulmon Dis 2014;9: 413.

36. Yokoba M, Ichikawa T, Takakura A, et al. Aminophylline increases respiratory muscle activity during hypercapnia in humans. Pulm Pharmacol Ther 2015; 30:96–101.

37. Anttalainen U, Saaresranta T, Vahlberg T, et al. Short-term medroxyprogesterone acetate in postmenopausal women with sleep-disordered breathing: a placebo-controlled, randomized, double-blind, parallel-group study. Menopause 2014;21(4):361–8.

Printed and bound by CPI Group (UK) Ltd, Croydon, CR0 4YY

03/10/2024

01040383-0009